Mental Health Aspects of Community Health Nursing

Mental Health Aspects of Community Health Nursing

Carolyn Chambers Clark, R.N., Ed.D.

Formerly, Adjunct Assistant Professor
Pace University–Westchester
Graduate School of Nursing

Mental Health Nursing Consultant and Specialist
Nursing Service, Inc., Ridgewood, New Jersey
and Visiting Nurses of Northern Bergen County
Mahwah, New Jersey

McGraw-Hill Book Company

New York   St. Louis   San Francisco   Auckland   Bogotá   Düsseldorf
Johannesburg   London   Madrid   Mexico   Montreal   New Delhi
Panama   Paris   São Paulo   Singapore   Sydney   Tokyo   Toronto

Library of Congress Cataloging in Publication Data

Clark, Carolyn Chambers.
  Mental health aspects of community health
nursing.

    Includes index.
    1. Community health nursing—Psychological
aspects. 2. Nurse and patient. 3. Community
mental health services. I. Title. [DNLM:
1. Community health nursing. 2. Psychiatric
nursing. 3. Nurse-patient relations. WY106 C592m]
RT98.C53   610.73'43   78-4852
ISBN 0-07-011150-2

MENTAL HEALTH ASPECTS OF COMMUNITY HEALTH NURSING

1234567890 DODO 78321098

This book was set in Press Roman by Allen Wayne Technical Corp.
The editor was Sally Barhydt, and the production supervisor was Jeanne Selzam.
The cover was designed by Tana Klugherz.
R. R. Donnelley & Sons Company was printer and binder.

Contents

2

OBSERVATION AND COMMUNICATION GUIDES

3

CASE CONSULTATIONS AND DISCUSSIONS

4

CASE STUDIES FOR PRACTICE

5

SIMULATED SITUATIONS FOR PRACTICE

Preface

Mental Health Aspects of Community Health Nursing evolved from two sources. The first source was my 6 years of consultation experience with community health nurses from two visiting nurse services. During this time, I met with groups of nurses as well as with individual nurses. To these meetings, the participants brought questions of how to understand and deal with the mental health aspects of their relationships with clients.

Initially, I presented theory and concepts to the community health nurses using informal group discussion and lecture methods. As the concepts of anxiety, conflict, guilt, grief, depression, and suicide became more familiar, case studies, process recordings, and family observation guides were used to apply the theory and concepts that had been discussed. Gradually, content related to family systems, substance abuse, social learning, and change was added. Finally, a guide for presenting problematic situations for individual and group consultation was formulated. Through the use of this guide, the nurses were able to present problematic nurse-client interactions and to identify goals in collaboration with me and their peers. Nurses often asked that I visit a client's home with them to validate their impressions. At these times, a preconference was used at which two or more of us developed goals for the joint visit. After the visit had been made, a postconference was held to share observations and develop possible nursing approaches. All these processes are reflected in the format of this book.

The second source for the text was my experience as a teacher in a graduate nursing program that prepared family nurse practitioners. Student questions about working with clients and families centered on practical aspects of how to handle the initial home visit, and how to relate with people in a therapeutic way. These student questions and discussions provided most of the ideas for the simulated situations for practice as well as for the case studies centering around the school, hospital clinic, and unstructured health care settings such as the single-room occupancy hotel.* These two sources of experience and clinical data underscored for me the scope of interest of both the novice student and the seasoned practitioner in the mental health aspects of community health nursing.

The book follows the natural progression of my consultation experiences. *Mental Health Aspects of Community Health Nursing* has five parts: "Theory and Concepts," "Observation and Communication Guides," "Case Consultations and Discussions," "Case Studies for Practice," and "Simulated Situations for Practice."

In Part 1, "Theory and Concepts," nurses are made aware of how their own feelings and reactions influence the nurse-client relationship, and how the clients' internal and external situations influence the nurse-client relationship. The focus of this part is the nurse-client relationship, with special emphasis on the nurse-family relationship. Community health nurses have always worked with families, but many of their interpersonal approaches have been intuitive or have been based on experiences they have had in their own families. In this book, nurses are given substantial working principles and concepts based on communication, family change, and social learning theory. These principles and concepts will allow the nurse to use a more organized and problem-solving approach in working with clients and families.

The goal of Part 2, "Observation and Communication Guides," is to orient learners to meaningful ways to assess and record mental health aspects of their work with individuals and families. The guides have been developed in collaboration with and field-tested by community health nurses and student family nurse practitioners.

In Part 3, "Case Consultations and Discussions," the learner is presented with actual community health nursing situations that exemplify the theories and concepts contained in the theory section. One goal of this part is to help the nurse generalize theory to more than one nurse-client situation. Through this generalization process, it should become clear to the learner that, no matter

---

*Names used in case studies are fictitious. Some case material has been expanded, combined, or condensed in order to illustrate specific concepts.

what the client's compliant, core mental health concepts are applicable. Case studies have been selected to demonstrate the applicability of mental health concepts to long- and short-term illness processes, substance abuse, normal growth and developmental crises, and situational crises. Nursing problems and interventions have been identified for each case.

Part 4, "Case Studies for Practice," presents the learner with actual situations that may arise in their community health work. A structured discussion guide follows each case and allows the learner to begin to think through his or her own assessments and interventions.

In Part 5, "Simulated Situations for Practice" allow groups of learners to get a feel for interacting with clients and families without having to learn everything from real life clients. The simulations can decrease interviewer anxiety considerably and allow for practice and repractice in a relatively nonthreatening environment.

Clearly, the focus of this book is not the psychiatric client. In most cases, the community health nurse will be working with clients whose presenting complaint is a physical one. As a primary practitioner, the community health nurse is in an unusually good position to provide skilled mental health interventions that can prevent future health problems, intervene in current family interactions that are nonconstructive, and support current coping devices when alternate solutions are not available.

This book also attempts to speak to the problem of isolation, which plagues the independent practitioner in the community. Community health nurses have told me of their sense of isolation and of awesome responsibility, as well as of emotional entanglements with clients that probably result in part from infrequent administrative and peer support and infrequent supervision. Mental health consultation seems to decrease some of these difficulties, and therefore I have attempted to translate into writing what I have learned from working with these nurses. I hope that community health nurses who do not have consultation available to them will benefit from what I have written. The material presented in this book will hopefully assist those nurses who do have a consultant available to them to organize information and present it to their mental health consultant in a more effective manner. I would hope that mental health consultants would also read this book and profit from my experience.

This book can be used in a number of ways. The learner may proceed through it as it is presented. Or, the learner may choose to focus on a concept and select learning experiences that relate to that concept. For example, the learner may read Chapter 2 on anxiety, then learn about how anxiety is assessed through process recordings and the Mental Health Assessment and Family Observation Guide. Then the reader may choose a Case Consultation such as Case 6 and a Case Study for Practice such as Case 10 to reinforce what was just read. Finally, a simulated situation such as Simulation 1 or Simulation 6 can provide the learner with actual practice in anxiety-reducing techniques for self and client.

To date, there is no other text that focuses on the mental health aspects of community health nursing. Most texts are oriented to the physical care aspects of community nursing or are collections of writings that do not seem to provide an orderly progression for the learner. *Mental Health Aspects of Community Health Nursing* brings a new integration of techniques and a framework for the treatment of the whole person. Some of the other strengths of this text are:

1 Behavioral objectives are tied to content and review questions.
2 There is an in-depth focus on the nurse and his or her reactions and what can be done to change them.
3 Theory is tied to practice through clinical examples, case studies, and simulated practice exercises.
4 In addition to being a basic text, the book can be used as a reference source whenever problematic nurse-client relationships occur.
5 Although a great deal of theory is presented, it has been organized in a highly readable way and in an easily digested style.
6 The problem-solving approach allows the learner to use nursing process.

This book is meant to be used by learners on a number of different levels. It can be used as a supplemental or additional text with other community health nursing texts in a baccalaureate nursing program. It could also be used in graduate nursing programs in community health, mental health, or family nurse practitioner programs. Graduate nurses in community health settings may find it a useful reference source. Nurses who wish to serve as consultants to other nurses regarding mental health aspects of practice could also benefit from this book. Supervisors and administrators of community health nurses may find value in the text.

I would like to acknowledge the assistance of the staffs of the two community health nursing agencies with which I am associated. I would especially like to thank Ms. Rita DeCotiis, Director of Nursing Service, Inc., and Ms. Joan Schroeder, Director of Visiting Nurses of Northern Bergen County. In addition, special thanks are due to Ms. Florence Soa and Ms. Mary Lowry for the use of process recording materials.

I also wish to thank the students in the Graduate School of Nursing at Pace University–Westchester who provided me with ideas for case studies as well as stimulating discussion.

Carolyn Chambers Clark

Part One

Theory and Concepts

Chapter 1

Health–Illness Relationships

LEARNING OBJECTIVES

When you finish this chapter, you should be able to:

- Identify how the client's perception of health and illness may influence nursing care
- Identify factors that can influence the client's ability to achieve homeostasis
- List factors that contribute to the acceptance of the sick role

Nurses are sometimes prone to zero in on the physical aspects of care and neglect the interplay between mind and body. How family members evaluate and react to mental or bodily changes is influenced by social, cultural, and environmental factors. Thus, you must be cognizant of the interplay of all variables that affect the client or family.

THE HOLISTIC APPROACH

A *holistic approach* to nursing care is one that attempts to consider the whole person, not merely the mind or the body. When using such an approach, you will try to understand how physiological, social, and cultural processes interrelate (Folta and Deck, 1965). A person will then be viewed as an open system when there is a continuous interchange between the internal environment of that person and the external environment of people, places, and things (Sutterly and Donnelly, 1973). People are thus actors as well as reactors; they create changes in their environment as well as react to changes within it. If you use this holistic approach, you assume that any function or malfunction of either mind or body will affect changes in the other.

Although this tenet is accepted intellectually by most nurses, it is not unusual to hear a remark such as, "Mr. Adams says he's in pain, but it's all in his mind." According to the holistic approach, pain is neither in the mind nor in the body. Pain is an experience that is influenced by anatomical and physiological factors (such as body build and stress to pressure points) and by mental or interpersonal factors (such as level of anxiety and previous experience with pain) as well as by social and cultural factors (such as definitions of pain and learned ways to express pain).

A holistic approach also includes an examination, with the client, of his or her perception of health and illness. All cultural groups and subgroups have ways to evaluate what is health and what is illness (Parsons, 1972). For example, the symptom of seeing things may be labelled as a hallucination by middle-class white Americans, but it may be regarded as a sign of holiness or as an indication of healing powers in Indian or Spanish subcultures. If you assume your values are the same as your clients' you are not using a holistic approach.

In order to define health and illness it is necessary to consider meaning. Whatever symptoms or signs may mean to you, these same symptoms and signs may have different meanings for clients or their families. Likewise, some people may define themselves as ill, yet not view medical or nursing care as necessary. For example, some ethnic groups are more likely to rely on folk medicine or family care than to seek out medical or nursing care.

Other groups may refuse to define themselves as ill because of the connotation illness has for them. For example, Christian Scientists are convinced that bodily illness is a result of negative thinking and loss of faith. When the Christian Scientist defines him- or herself as ill, he or she runs the risk of losing the support of friends and family. Table 1-1 attempts to help you to assess the interrelationships of physiological and sociocultural processes.

HOMEOSTASIS

Homeostasis is a term that is used to describe the healthy, relatively stable state where no undue imbalance exists (Miller, 1969). An imbalance, or unstable state, can occur when people are unable to adapt. *Adaptation* is a process whereby people regulate both what goes on inside them and in their immediate external

Table 1-1 Assessing the Client's Perception of Health and Illness

Assessment area	Questions to ask during the assessment
Understanding symptom meaning	What did you think was happening when you first noticed the symptom?
	What clues do you have that you're healthy?
	What do you notice about yourself that tells you that you may be ill?
Understanding the health care system	Where do you go for help when you feel ill?
	Have you found nurses (doctors) to be helpful to you in the past?
	Which agency procedures do you find difficult (humiliating, frustrating, unclear)?
Sociocultural influences	How do you think your family feels about your health?
	How do you feel about the state of your health?
	What helps you when you're in pain?
	What do you think caused your health (illness)?
	What comments have you heard about the state of your health from people of your religion?

environment meaningfully and successfully. The more adaptive or flexible people are, the healthier they are. People who constantly use withdrawal from confrontations as an adaptive maneuver are probably less healthy than those who sometimes withdraw and who at other times assert themselves. Likewise, people who have money, education, or power may find it easier to adapt to a recession than those who do not have these assets. Similarly, some people may receive more support from family, friends, or professional helpers, and are thus more capable of adapting than those with the same condition who do not have these supports. For example, a husband who has recently retired could be searching for a new role. This change in his available free time could lead him to develop a whole new role, to try to supplant his wife in her role, or to become depressed. If and how the man's wife, friends, and professional helpers provide support for him will influence how well he adapts to his new life-style.

All behavior can be assumed to be meaningful and to be need- or goal-directed. Some patient or family behavior may appear at first to be not only ineffective, but also meaningless or discordant with your goals. Although you may know the relevant nursing goals for increasing patient independence and action, these goals may at times be in opposition to patient or family goals. This may be especially the case when the patient is dying. Frequently, health professionals see their role as preventing illness and promoting health. Thus, when the person is dying, you may feel frustrated and angry and may carry out desperate measures to over-come your own feelings of helplessness (Sitzman, 1974).

For example, in a case conference to discuss a person who was dying, several community health nurses reported that the dying person cloistered herself away in a second-floor bedroom and refused to see any friends or many family members. The nurses spent a great deal of discussion time challenging each other's nursing goals as being not supportive of the patient's independent actions. When the mental health nursing consultant suggested that perhaps the patient was further along in accepting her death than they were, the nurses were able to use a framework where what was happening in the family was viewed as a homeo-static balance in which every family member had found a way to adapt to the event of impending death. Since the loosening of interpersonal relationships is considered by Kübler-Ross (1970) to be a normal process as death approaches, this framework added additional meaning to the discussion and led to a change in nursing goals.

A breakdown in homeostatic devices can occur on a number of levels. Wher-ever the breakdown occurs, other levels of functioning will be affected. For example, it is accepted that potential invading organisms are present in our external environment all the time. It is usually only when stressors such as inadequate nutrition, high level of anxiety, or genetic defect are combined with the available invading organisms that a homeostatic breakdown occurs and illness results. Suppose that the illness in question is multiple sclerosis. The per-son may then become quite angry and depressed about his or her debilitating condition, and may consider (and even commit) suicide. Likewise, the diagnosis and subsequent emotional response of the patient will affect his or her family and friends. As debilitation increases, family members will have to adapt so as to provide more physical care for the patient. One adaptational device the family may use is to call in the community health nurse.

Homeostatic imbalances can also begin at the emotional level. A community health nurse was asked to visit a woman who had a lifelong history of withdrawal and a depressive style of living. The woman was suddenly faced with the depar-ture of her oldest son from the family; shortly thereafter she developed symptoms of ulcerative colitis. Her anger and rage had evidently turned inward and she was literally stewing in her own juices. The ulcerations became so acute that an ileos-tomy was performed. The community health nurse noted that the family mem-bers showed signs of reacting to their mother's physical and emotional changes. The oldest daughter, Rita, suffered an increase in allergic reactions and gained 20 pounds over a 3-month period. The patient's husband began to drink more and to work late at the office, and their sexual relationship ended. In this case, what began as a normal family crisis led to a strong emotional and physical reac-tion on the part of the mother and to subsequent physical and emotional re-sponses in other family members as they reacted to increased family stress. The mother was unable to accept her ileostomy, and family members also showed signs of disgust and revulsion related to stomal functioning. The mother became more depressed and took to her bed (a tactic she had employed after the birth of each of her children). At this point, the community health nurse referred the family to the psychiatric mental health nurse for counseling. Table 1-2 shows the nursing problems the psychiatric mental health nurse worked on with this family.

Physiological mechanisms of homeostasis have been well documented (Selye, 1976), but there is less agreement about what psychological variables are important to study, and when they are identified (Sitzman, 1974) they are often difficult to measure. Further complicating this difficulty may be your own need to have families act on the information and advice you have given them. Thus, not always being able to see immediate results from a therapeutic relationship and needing to have the family's approval and full cooperation can upset rather than restore homeostatic balance because then family members must not only cope with the effect of their stressors, but also use valuable energy to please you.

THE SICK ROLE AND THE DIFFERENT ROLE

Health used to be thought of as the absence of illness. Now, how we perceive illness and wellness is considered to be an important element in our definition of health or illness. Illness can be viewed as a response to social pressures. When the patient escapes into illness, he or she is relieved of role responsibilities such as that of family member, wage earner, and religious person (Parsons, 1972).

Table 1-2 The Psychiatric Mental Health Nurse's Goals and Interventions with a Family Where One Member Has an Ileostomy

Type of session	Goals	Interventions
Individual	1 Resolve grief	Direct patient to discuss thoughts and feelings about ileostomy and son's leaving
	2 Strengthen coping responses	a Do not respond to complaints or pleas to talk to other family members for her except to encourage family sessions b Comment on positive coping attempts
Family	3 Open up communication channels	Show family members how to talk with one another
	4 Support coping behaviors	Point out family behaviors that are healthy as they occur
	5 Resolve grief	Assist family members to discuss reactions to family changes

Before they accept the sick role, people often use familiar coping devices. Frantic escapes such as working overtime or excessive socializing may be observed. One community health nurse reported that a female patient whom she was treating for ostomy leakage had a husband who had recently been diagnosed as having glaucoma and who had begun to stay away from home more and more and to play poker with "the boys" more than he ever had before. Such behavior certainly seemed to indicate the man's reluctance to accept the sick role. Instead of coping directly with his condition, he tried to use familiar devices such as playing cards as a way of dealing with his vision loss.

At the same time people are trying to use familiar coping devices, they may also be searching for an explanation of their symptoms. Some questions that may cross their minds when unfamiliar symptoms or signs occur are:

Is there something seriously wrong because I can't remember people's names?
Is that one hallucination that I had a sign of madness?
Does that constant headache mean I have a brain tumor?
Does that bleeding mean I have cancer?
Does leakage from my stoma mean I'll have to have more surgery?

In some cultural groups or subgroups it may be perfectly acceptable for people to completely treat their own bodily signs or symptoms. In other cultural groups, the symptomatic person may turn to family or friends for reassurance. If they discount the symptoms, the symptomatic person will be less likely to seek outside help. If, on the other hand, self-treatment is ineffective and family and friends exert pressure on the person to seek help, medical or nursing assistance may be sought.

There seem to be a number of factors that interrelate and influence whether a person accepts or refuses to accept the sick role. One factor is the number and persistence of symptoms. A minor symptom that occurs once or twice is not likely to be taken seriously by most people. Another factor is the person's ability to recognize symptoms or signs. If the person is not aware that blackouts may be a sign of alcoholism or of rising blood pressure, he or she may not seek help simply because of lack of information. Another factor is the perceived degree of social or physical disability. In some age groups such as the elderly, decreased sociability and increased physical disability are the norm, and, therefore, may not be treated with alarm. In the case of a young adult, decreased sociability and increased physical disability may have a major effect on his or her wage-earning ability and thus may be treated with more concern by others than would a similar condition in an elderly person.

Cultural learnings are another factor that influence whether a person accepts the sick role. In some cultures people are taught to grin and bear pain or unusual symptoms. Other cultural groups teach their members to complain loudly and to seek help when certain body areas are affected.

A major influence on whether the sick role is accepted is the degree of disruption that the illness causes in the sufferer's life-style. If a person can no longer carry on activities of daily living, friends and family may pressure him or her to ask for professional assistance. Since these factors interrelate, you need to assess each of them for each client.

Once the sick role is adopted, it may not be easily given up. Some psychiatric patients or people with chronic physical illnesses may adopt a lifelong sick role. They may view their role as being dependent on others to maintain their activities of daily life. The sick role can be seen as an exchange process where freedom and control are exchanged for care, protection, and freedom from responsibility.

One community health nurse was asked to visit a woman who had been hit by a car and who had sustained multiple lacerations and fractures. Long after her discharge from a rehabilitation center, the person remained in a wheelchair, refused to cooperate and do muscle-strengthening exercises, and showed many indirect signs of unresolved grief and refusal to resume the well role. The nurse referred the patient and her family to the psychiatric mental health nurse because she felt that the family was subtly discouraging the patient from being more independent and from expressing her anger directly.

For people with chronic conditions or long-term disabilities, the important distinction you can communicate to them is that they are not sick, but that they are permanently different. As long as a person who is at the highest level of physical functioning possible has a self-view as a sick person, he or she will have expectations of getting well and may look for cures rather than concentrating on adapting to a change in life-style.

One community health nurse worked with a 40-year-old woman who had multiple sclerosis. At a certain point, the woman remained for several years in a period of remission of her physical symptoms, although she was by then in a wheelchair and required an indwelling catheter. She had learned to transfer herself from wheelchair to easy chair, but seemed highly anxious about her condition and alternated between transferring herself and refusing to do so. She seemed to think a cure might be discovered, and at those times she refused to transfer herself. When the community health nurse began to feel frustrated with this person, she referred her to the psychiatric mental health nursing specialist. Table 1-3 shows the nursing problems the psychiatric mental health nurse worked on with this family.

BIOLOGICAL RHYTHMS AND HEALTH

A person's level of health changes week by week and even hour by hour. People establish their own patterns or body rhythms. A study of body rhythms explains why people are more susceptible to infection or emotional upset at certain times of the day. Body rhythm explains why people perform at high or low levels at different times in their work or nonwork day. An upset in biological rhythm

Table 1-3   The Psychiatric Mental Health Nurse's Goals and Interventions with a Family in Which One Member Has Multiple Sclerosis

Type of session	Goals	Interventions
Individual	1 Decrease anxiety	Remain present and actively listen
	2 Resolve grief	Direct patient to discuss thoughts and feelings about having multiple sclerosis
	3 Strengthen coping responses	Point out healthy behaviors
	4 Teach adaptive behaviors	a Teach parenting skills b Assist with behavior rehearsal in social situations
Family	1 Resolve grief	Assist all family members to discuss thoughts, feelings, and changes that have occurred as a result of mother's debility
	2 Teach adaptive behaviors	a Reinforce verbalizations b Teach family members to develop behavioral contracts
	3 Improve communication between husband and wife	Use structured exercises to help spouses practice more effective communication

often signals an illness process. For example, unusual changes in bowel or sleep habits or sudden emotional flare-ups can signal an upset in homeostasis via body rhythms.

You can assess your own and your client's body rhythms in the following areas: activity/rest, food/fluid, elimination, interpersonal mood, and symptoms. Both you and your clients can learn more about individual body rhythms by keeping a chart over a period of time that records body rhythm changes. For an example of a partial body rhythm assessment chart, see Table 1-4; for the assessment to be most useful, it must be charted over a period of several weeks (Luce, 1971).

Besides charting body rhythms, people can also learn more about their body functioning through biofeedback. *Biofeedback* is the information a person receives about his or her body. *Biofeedback training* is a method by which people learn to tune into their body functions and even to control them. Although much of biofeedback training takes place in laboratories with monitoring equipment, you can apply the essential principles to your work with some additional assistance from a mental health nursing specialist.

For example, you can teach a client to tune into body tension that often occurs in chest and neck musculature. Such heightened states of muscular

Table 1-4 Body Rhythm Assessment Chart

Date	Assessments
12/1	Slept: from _____ p.m. to _____ p.m. a.m. a.m. Napped: from _____ p.m. to _____ p.m. a.m. a.m. Concentrated best at: _____ Most active at: _____ Ate breakfast at: _____ Ate lunch at: _____ Ate supper at: _____ Snacked at: _____ Had bowel movement at: _____ type: _____ Urinated at: _____ type: _____ Felt depressed at: _____ (time) Felt happy at: _____ Felt foggy or was unable to think clearly at: _____ Felt tired at: _____ Felt sensitive at: _____ Felt like being alone at: _____ Felt like being with others at: _____ Had the following symptoms at: _____
12/2	Slept: from _____ p.m. to _____ p.m. a.m. a.m. Napped: from _____ p.m. to _____ p.m. a.m. a.m.

tension can lead to backaches and headaches, as well as contribute to decreased general circulation and respiratory difficulty. Increased chronic tension in musculature can lead to postural difficulties, insomnia, and greater susceptibility to injury from falls or accidents. People can learn to be aware of their body tension levels and decrease them accordingly (Ornstein, 1972).

SUMMARY

A holistic approach to clients and their problems includes an assessment of how physiological, social, and cultural processes interrelate. Homeostasis is a term that describes the healthy, relatively stable state where no undue imbalance exists. People with chronic conditions can be assisted to higher levels of wellness by being encouraged to view themselves as different rather than as sick. Health is an ever-changing process that can be assessed via biological rhythms and biofeedback.

PRACTICE EXERCISES

1 Pair off with another person. Ask one another the questions listed in Table 1-1.
2 Chart your own body rhythms for a month using the assessment areas listed in Table 1-4.

REVIEW*

Multiple-Choice Questions

1 A client's perception of health and illness can influence nursing care in which of the following way(s)?
   a The client may not seek the services of a nurse if sociocultural factors dictate against his or her taking such an action.
   b The client may need to know more about and better understand the meaning of his or her symptoms.
   c All clients will demonstrate similar outward reactions to their symptoms.
   d Biofeedback will be provided.
2 Which of the following factors can influence the client's ability to achieve homeostasis?
   a ability to adapt
   b amount of education, money, social supports
   c the nurse's need to be liked or approved of
   d combining both the sick role and the different role

Listing

List factors that contribute to the acceptance of the sick role.

_____

_____

_____

REFERENCES

Abram, H. S., ed. 1967. *Psychological aspects of surgery*. Boston: Little, Brown.
Adams, J., and Lindemann, E. 1974. Coping with longterm disability. In *Coping and adaptation*, ed. G. Coelho, pp. 127–138. New York: Basic Books.
Clark, C. C. 1977. *Nursing concepts and processes*. Albany: Delmar.
Folta, J., and Deck, E., eds. 1965. *A sociological framework for patient care*. New York: Wiley.
Kübler-Ross, E. 1970. *Death and dying*. New York: Macmillan.
Luce, G. 1971. *Body time*. New York: Pantheon.

*Answers to the end-of-chapter review exercises will be found in the Answer Key (see p. 261).

Miller, J. 1969. Living systems; basic concepts. In *General systems theory and psychiatry*, eds. W. Gray, F. Duhl, and N. Rizzo, pp. 51–133. Boston: Little, Brown.

Moos, R. H., ed. 1977. *Coping with physical illness.* New York: Plenum.

Ornstein, R. 1972. *The psychology of consciousness.* San Francisco: Freeman.

Parsons, T. 1972. Definitions of health and illness in light of American values and social structure. In *Patients, physicians and illness.* 2d ed., ed. E. Jaco, pp. 97–117. New York: Free Press.

Selye, H. 1976. *The stress of life.* rev. ed. New York: McGraw-Hill.

Silverman, S. 1970. *Psychological cues in forecasting physical illness.* New York: Appleton-Century-Crofts.

Sitzman, J. 1974. Psychosomatic disorders. In *New dimensions in mental health-psychiatric nursing*, eds. M. E. Kalkman and A. J. Davis. pp. 417–450. New York: McGraw-Hill.

Sutterly, D., and Donnelly, G. 1973. *Perspectives in human development: nursing throughout the life cycle.* Philadelphia: Lippincott.

Chapter 2

Anxiety

LEARNING OBJECTIVES

When you finish this chapter, you should be able to:

- Define anxiety
- List four sources of anxiety
- List four levels of anxiety
- Match patient and family coping devices with appropriate examples
- Identify nursing interventions that are useful in dealing with different levels of anxiety

Anxiety is a feeling of unexplained discomfort that can occur when people are faced with the unexpected, the embarrassing, the unfamiliar, the disapproval of others, or their own unmet needs. Anxiety occurs whenever there is a threat to interpersonal security (Sullivan, 1953).

MEANING AND SOURCES OF ANXIETY

All people experience anxiety in varying degrees throughout their lifetimes. Nurses as well as patients feel anxious. Being alive and interested means that there is at least a mild level of anxiety present. An anxious patient or client can cause you to become anxious. This occurs because anxiety is a feeling that is learned and experienced in relation to other people. As infants, all of us have most likely been held by an anxious mother. It was at that time that we first probably realized that all was not right. It was impossible to realize then that that unexplained feeling of discomfort was the feeling of anxiety. As we grew older, feelings of anxiety were apt to occur when a situation was embarrassing, unfamiliar, or when our self-esteem was threatened. Anxiety can occur whether you work with a family in their familiar home setting, or whether you see the family in an agency setting. Being familiar with common sources of anxiety can help you to zero in on these sources and to use nursing approaches that promote mental health in others. By decreasing anxiety in yourself and in others you will increase the energy available to you for nursing care.

Perhaps the most common source of anxiety is the unexpected occurrence. Expecting one situation to occur, and then finding an entirely different one can be a perplexing, if not a threatening, experience. Suppose you want the patient to live, but he or she prefers to die? Suppose you expect the patient to take his or her medication, but the patient refuses? Suppose you try to teach a patient how to walk with crutches, but the patient falls down in the middle of your lesson? Suppose you have a nursing care plan all written out on the patient's chart, but the patient says, "I don't need your help; I can manage myself"? Suppose you give the patient's family explicit directions for patient care, and then the family ignores them? Suppose you expect the doctor to share information with you about the patient, but the doctor never returns your phone calls? Each of these situations is one where what you expected to happen did not happen. Therefore, each of these situations can end in your experiencing the discomfort of anxiety.

Patients or clients can feel anxious when you behave in a way they did not expect. Suppose the patient wants you to cure his cancer, while your goal is to help the patient rest comfortably? Suppose the patient wants to talk with you about death and dying, but you want to give her a bedbath? Suppose the patient expects to be transferred slowly from his bed to a chair, and you whisk him away in a Hoyer lift? Each of these situations has the potential for creating anxiety in the patient because he or she expected one thing to happen, and something different occurred.

Another source of anxiety is when the client asks you an embarrassing question. If you happen to be a young nurse who is struggling to act professionally, the question, "How old are you, anyway?" can lead to anxiety. If you are a nurse who is unsure of your relationship with the opposite sex, a question such as, "Why aren't you married yet?" can evoke anxiety. If you have difficulty setting limits on impossible patient demands, the question, "Why can't you give me a shampoo and set?" may lead to an anxious feeling. Clients or patients may be embarrassed by different situations. Some may experience anxiety when given their first bedbath, when having their new incision or drain peered at by you, or when asked to buy equipment they cannot afford. At other times, you or a client might be unsure of your appearance, and think that you are unattractive; when someone comments about your physical appearance, anxiety can occur. Since what is embarrassing for you may not be embarrassing for other nurses or clients, it will be helpful for you to think about and jot down situations that you find embarrassing. Becoming aware of anxiety-provoking situations is the first step toward handling them more effectively.

Another source of anxiety for both you and the patient is the unfamiliar situation. The first time you enter someone's home, you will no doubt feel anxious. Some thoughts that may cross your mind are: "Will I like this person?" "Will this person like me and see me as helpful?" "Will this person slam the door in my face?" On the other side of the door, the patient is probably experiencing some anxiety as he or she thinks: "Will the nurse like me?" "Will he or she be critical of my housekeeping?" and maybe, "Will the nurse hurt or expose me in some way?"

Both you and the patient can experience anxiety if you anticipate the other's disapproval. If you are told by a patient you like and respect, "You didn't do that right," anxiety can result. If an instructor or supervisor tells you, "Your nursing care is poor," anxiety can result. If you let a client know through your words or actions that you think he or she is a bad person for not obeying you, that person will probably feel anxious.

When you or the patient has an unmet need for oxygen, food and fluid, activity, rest, reparation of damage, avoidance of injury, elimination of waste, or interpersonal relationships, anxiety can result. When you skip lunch or miss sleep, you can feel more irritable and anxious with others. Clients or patients who have difficulty breathing or moving may feel anxious because of their unmet needs.

A basic interpersonal need that can lead to anxiety if it is unmet is the need to be respected or recognized. The patient may show disrespect or nonrecognition by saying thing such as, "You better ask the doctor; I don't think you know what you're doing" or "You don't know what you're talking about." Such statements can be experienced by you as challenges to your professional ability. Patients, too, can feel anxious when you are too friendly too soon, or when you do not ask the patient for an opinion on his or her care.

There is a special form of anxiety called *performance anxiety* that can plague both you and the patient. Performance anxiety is likely to turn up whenever people are unable to perform in the way they would like to perform. The first time you enter a patient's home you may feel anxious in anticipation of how you will perform nursing care. Some performance anxiety thoughts that you may have are: "Can I do the procedure correctly and smoothly?" "Will the patient know I'm unsure of my ability to perform this care?"

Even an experienced nurse can experience performance anxiety when trying a new or modified procedure with a patient. Performance anxiety can also creep in when you feel intimidated by or confused about the patient's behavior. When people speak angrily to you, cry, or continue to become more debilitated, you may be threatened and subsequently feel anxious. Such situations may lead you to think, "Did I do something wrong?" "How can I work smoothly and efficiently when I'm being watched?" and "If I were a good nurse, she wouldn't be getting worse." When any of these thoughts enter your head, they are likely to influence your effectiveness as a nurse because anxiety will interfere with your ability to function properly.

Patients, too, can experience performance anxiety. Any serious illness leads to a decrease in functioning in physiological, social, and occupational areas. The client can experience anxiety because he or she knows performance has decreased in some area. Patients who are extremely weak or dependent, or who are required to learn new or difficult procedures can feel anxious until they are secure in performing a task. For example, patients with multiple sclerosis report a high degree of anxiety about their ability to move steadily without muscle spasm. This anxiety about performing can add to the patient's stress level, and increase the possibility of further muscle spasm. Table 2-1 details some sources of anxiety in the nurse-patient relationship.

LEVELS OF ANXIETY

Your level of anxiety can change in relation to the patient's level and vice versa. A patient who was highly anxious prior to your arrival can become less anxious just by being with you if you remain calm. Or, you can be calm and relaxed at the beginning of a day's work, but suddenly become irritable and fatigued after a brief encounter with a dying, angry, or crying patient.

Although anxiety probably occurs on a continuum that extends from no anxiety to panic it is useful to think of levels or categories of anxiety for purposes of assessment and intervention. An anxiety level that dips below mild anxiety or rises above moderate anxiety usually leads to less effective functioning. Different levels of anxiety can be assessed by observing physiological cues and social behaviors (Peplau, 1963).

Mild Anxiety

When you or your client is mildly anxious, you are alert and interested in what is happening around you. The person who is in the mild anxiety state is able to use all of his or her senses to the utmost. The sensory information that you receive from the environment is seen, heard, felt, tasted, and sniffed in an open and interested fashion. Communication with other people is clear and direct. Feelings of being threatened by others or by situations or procedures are minimal.

When you or the patient is mildly anxious, there is sufficient body muscle

Table 2-1   Sources of Anxiety

Source	Examples
The unexpected	*The nurse expects:* the client to take his medication, but he refuses the members of the family to follow his or her directions, but they refuse *The client expects:* the nurse to talk with her about her fears, but he or she makes the bed instead to be transferred smoothly and slowly to her bed, but instead is moved quickly and jerkily
The embarrassing	*The nurse can be embarrassed when:* the patient asks his or her age a client teases about his or her weight *The patient can be embarrassed when:* she is examined by a male nurse he is examined by a female nurse
The unfamiliar	*The nurse can feel anxious when:* he or she tries a new procedure he or she visits a family for the first time *The patient can feel anxious when:* he is asked to try a new behavior the nurse visits for the first time
Having to perform when unsure of oneself	*The nurse can feel unsure when:* he or she is faced with a care situation that has previously turned out badly the patient gets worse despite effective nursing care *The client can feel unsure when:* she is intimidated or confused she is feeling dependent or debilitated
Unmet needs	*The nurse can feel unexplained discomfort when:* the client challenges his or her ability he or she is unable to eat a leisurely lunch *The patient can feel unexplained discomfort when:* he cannot move the nurse calls him by the wrong name

tone to carry out vital body functions, but there is not enough to lead to tension or fatigue. Vital signs are stable, pupils of the eyes are dilated and open to incoming information, and speech is moderate in pace and clear in enunciation.

When both you and the patient are mildly anxious, the stage is best set for learning to occur. It is at this point that you will be most successful in trying to teach the patient. Table 2-2 lists some questions that you can ask yourself about

Table 2-2 Mild Anxiety Assessment Questions

Questions for the nurse	Questions for the patient or client
Do I feel alert, open, and accepting of what is happening around me?	Does the patient or client seem to be hearing, seeing, and sensing the situation?
Am I turned toward the patient, and am I maintaining steady eye contact?	Is the patient turned toward me and is he maintaining steady eye contact?
Do I have good muscle tone or am I tense?	Does the patient have good muscle tone or is he tense?
Do my gestures and body movements seem natural and relaxed?	Do the patient's gestures and body movements seem natural and relaxed?
Do my pulse and respiration seem slow and steady?	Do the patient's pulse and respiration seem slow and steady?
Is my speech moderate in pace and am I enunciating clearly?	Is the patient's speech moderate in pace and is he enunciating clearly?

your own or the patient's anxiety. If all or most of the answers are "yes," mild anxiety is probably present.

Moderate Anxiety

A greater degree of tension and anxiety can be noted in the moderate level of anxiety. Learning can still occur at this level. In fact, intricate tasks that require focused attention may be best accomplished at this level. A narrowing of attention occurs in both you and the patient at the moderate anxiety level; neither of you will be as able to sense all that is happening around you as you normally would be because you will be focusing your attention on a task or procedure.

Body tension increases as you or the patient strain to accomplish the task. Some perspiring of the palms or underarms may occur. Pulse and respiration may speed up as you experience feelings of exhilaration or exert yourself in the course of completing the task. Fatigue and increased body tension can lead to tension headaches. The rate of speech may increase. Each of you will probably have your own signals of increasing anxiety. You can begin to notice what your individual signals are: some people get butterflies in the stomach, tightness in the throat, and so on. You can also observe the patient for signs that he or she is becoming more nervous or upset. Table 2-3 lists some questions that can be used to assess moderate anxiety. If all or most of the answers are "yes," moderate anxiety is probably present. In addition to observing the patient, you can also ask him questions such as, "How do you know when you're upset; what happens inside you?"

Somewhere between moderate and severe anxiety, you and the patient begin to narrow your perception even further so that you notice only parts of the total situation. For example, if you feel threatened by the patient who says he or she

Table 2-3 Moderate Anxiety Assessment Questions

Questions for the nurse	Questions for the patient or client
Do I seem to be focusing on a specific task or topic of conversation?	Is the patient or client narrowing her attention in order to complete a task?
Is my body tension increasing?	Is the patient's body tension increasing?
Am I straining or maintaining one body position for more than a few minutes?	Is the patient straining or maintaining one body position for more than a few minutes?
Do I feel exhilarated or as if I'm exerting myself to accomplish the task?	Does the patient seem to be straining to accomplish the task?
Do I have sweaty palms or underarms in a cool room?	Is the patient beginning to perspire even though the room is cool?
Do I notice my usual signs of increasing anxiety such as tension headache, butterflies in my stomach, or tightening in my throat?	Is the patient showing signs of behavior that you have observed to be indicative of increasing anxiety?

wants to die, you may hear the patient's words but may not pay attention to the tone of voice, body posture, or gestures that accompany the words. In fact, you may only hear part of what is said, and you may choose to hear only what you want to hear. Likewise, when you tell a patient that he or she must submit to a painful procedure, that patient may hear nothing that you say after you indicated that the procedure will be painful. When both you and the patient are at this level of anxiety, neither of you is fully comprehending the other.

Severe Anxiety

When either you or the patient is at the severe anxiety level, you cannot perceive whole situations or experiences. It is not always possible to predict what situations will lead to severe anxiety. What is threatening to you may not be threatening to another nurse or patient. Some situations that commonly produce severe anxiety are the unexpected death of a patient, being fired, or addressing a large audience without previous experience in public speaking.

Likewise, different patients find different experiences threatening. For some patients, being told that they need surgery, that they are dying, or that they will be sent to a nursing home will set off a severe anxiety reaction.

At the severe anxiety level, no learning is possible. When you or the patient is severely anxious, only automatic, repetitive behaviors are apt to occur. You may only be aware of feeling wooden, strange, or unreal at the time you are experiencing severe anxiety. It is only later, when anxiety has decreased, that you can begin to figure out what led up to the anxiety attack. The ability to trace back the source of the anxiety can be a very helpful skill that can lead to your experiencing fewer episodes of severe anxiety in the future. It is best not to try to do this with the patient if either you or the patient is at this level of anxiety since no learning will occur and you will merely waste your energy.

The attention span of you or the patient is short when either of you is experiencing severe anxiety. You tend to focus on small details of a situation or on scattered, seemingly unconnected details. After an experience where you were at this level of anxiety, you may have vivid recollections that the patient wore an emerald ring, but you may have little recall of what was said or done. Or, you may remember fragments of an interchange, but you may not remember what happened during the time you tried to restrain a combative patient.

If you are experiencing mild or moderate anxiety, and the patient is severely anxious, you can still observe behavioral clues to the patient's level of anxiety. One of the things you will notice is a tendency to jump from one seemingly unconnected topic to another; for example, the patient might talk about the weather, his mean mother, purple tulips, and a murder in a short period of time without bothering to tell you how these ideas are connected. The speech of severely anxious people may seem puzzling and bewildering to you. What has happened is that the logical connections between topics of events are missing. In usual social conversation, the speaker tells the listener how to interpret what is being said. For example, the speaker may say, "This weather reminds me of when I was a kid and how my mother used to keep me indoors when it rained. She sure was mean." In other instances of conversation, the speaker lets the listener know how to take what is being said by his or her tone of voice, facial expressions, or bodily gestures. These nonverbal clues can tell the listener such things as: "I'm serious now" "This is a joke" or "I'm feeling exploited." When the speaker is severely anxious, he or she cannot make these logical connections and cannot give these clues to the listener. This is why you feel at a loss to interpret the actions and words of a severely anxious person.

Severe anxiety may reveal itself in physiological cues. You or the client may not experience the discomfort of severe anxiety, but you may perspire profusely, and have diarrhea or a frequent urge to urinate. Your breathing may become shallow and rapid. Speech is often fast, constant, loud, hesitant, or high-pitched. A patient could behave in a way that is so threatening to you that you may find yourself screeching at him or her. When you are severely anxious your own voice may sound distant, too loud, or as if someone else, not you, were speaking. Muscular tension is further increased, and tremors, shivers, and clenched fists are not unlikely to occur. Table 2-4 presents a list of severe anxiety assessment questions for both patient and nurse.

Panic

Panic places severe stress on a person. Long periods of panic can be so stressful that physiological functioning is paralyzed. In panic, you or the patient probably experience feelings of dread, terror, and unreality. Communication with others is so unclear, that it is almost impossible to understand.

Table 2-4 Severe Anxiety Assessment Questions

Questions for the nurse	Questions for the patient or client
Did I remember only vaguely most of what the patient said?	Did the patient seem not to hear what I said after a certain point in the visit?
Did any of the situations that create severe anxiety in me occur?	Did any of the situations occur that might lead to severe anxiety in the patient?
Did I feel as though I were acting in an automatic, unreal, or rote way?	Did the patient repeat words or tasks?
Did I have difficulty focusing on what the patient said or did?	Did the patient have difficulty focusing on what I said or did?
Did I remember only one small aspect of the visit?	Did the patient's speech bewilder and confuse me?
Did I perspire profusely, have diarrhea, or urinate frequently?	Did the patient perspire profusely, have diarrhea, or urinate frequently?
Were my respirations shallow and rapid?	Were the patient's respirations shallow and rapid?
Was my voice screechy, loud, too fast, constant, hesitant, or high-pitched?	Was the patient's speech too loud, fast, constant, hesitant, or high-pitched?
Did I shiver, tremble, or clench my fists?	Did the patient shiver, tremble, or clench his or her fists?

You will rarely experience panic or see a patient in panic. Catastrophic situations such as fires, floods, or massive loss of life may lead to panic in people who are not prepared for such situations. You could experience panic when taken by surprise by a highly threatening situation or event.

People experiencing acute psychotic episodes or hallucinogenic drug reactions may also experience panic. This is because highly threatening experiences that they had previously forgotten or repressed suddenly burst into their awareness. The breaking through of this highly threatening material can lead to the feelings of dread and terror associated with panic. (See Figure 2-1 for a listing of panic assessment questions.) Because anxiety is such an uncomfortable experience, many people cope with it by converting the discomfort they feel into more

Figure 2-1 Panic Assessment Questions

Is verbal communication nearly or completely incomprehensible?

Is a catastrophic situation occurring?

Is an acute psychotic episode occurring?

Is an hallucinogenic drug reaction occurring?

comfortable behaviors. Attack, withdrawal, somatization, and learning are four of the commonest ways to decrease anxiety.

HOW CLIENTS AND FAMILIES COPE WITH ANXIETY

The most common device for dealing with anxiety is to *attack* the other person. When a client or family member feels threatened, he or she can decrease discomfort by attacking other family members or you. Starting an argument, showing unreasonable anger, or subtly belittling the other person are all ways to decrease the discomfort of anxiety.

The client may think such thoughts as, "The nurse is better than I am; she is educated" "I'm afraid of being involved with the nurse" "I worry about being rejected by people" or "This new procedure scares me." Often, people may not even be aware of having this type of thought. Instead, anxiety is immediately converted into an attack on a family member or on you. Examples of such attacks include the following, "Be careful; you aren't doing that right" "Go away and don't come back!" "You're stupid; you don't know what you're saying" and "You better not try that without checking with the doctor first, dearie."

In some cases, two family members who have been attacking one another may turn on you if you attempt to take one or the other's side in an argument. When working with family members who do this, try to remember that this is their way of dealing with anxiety, and is probably not because they are angry with you. It is generally a good policy not to side with any family member, even the patient, unless you believe there is a chance of physical harm occurring.

Children can use an attacking form of intimidation with their parents when they feel anxious. They may say, "Bad Mommy" or "You're bad" when forced to go to school, enter unfamiliar situations, or perform in situations where they feel inferior or threatened.

Withdrawal is another way that patients and families cope with anxiety. Withdrawal is often used by people who fear becoming angry, or who fear really experiencing their feelings. Withdrawal can take a physical or an emotional form. Withdrawn people tend to make few complaints and interact infrequently with others. To you, the withdrawn person may seem to be doing all right. But in reality, that person may be highly anxious and may withdraw as a way of coping with anxious feelings. When depressed, the person may be quite anxious about him- or herself and the ability to function and be liked by others. In depression, there is a physical as well as an emotional or social withdrawal. The person may turn away from others, have unsteady eye contact, look drawn and dejected, and generally communicate through his or her body posture, "I am worthless, unlovable, and incompetent." Underneath this veneer of indifference and hopelessness may exist a great deal of anger that the depressed, withdrawn person is afraid of expressing.

Somatization is another way clients and families deal with anxiety. Through the process of somatization, anxiety is converted into physical symptoms. Anxiety can be converted into an increase in blood pressure, a tension headache, diarrhea, fatigue, or may be expressed in the form of other bodily symptoms. Those who use this method to avoid experiencing anxiety may do so quite automatically. Helping people to become aware that they are using somatization as a coping mechanism can be a long and difficult task. Sometimes you may see patients or family members looking outwardly calm at a time when anxiety on their part would be most expected. What you may fail to suspect is that complaints of hypertension, headache, diarrhea, or fatigue may actually be cues that, underneath it all, the person is anxious. Children who complain frequently of tummy aches or other illnesses may be highly anxious about some aspect of their school or home situation.

Learning is the most constructive way to channel the energy of anxiety. Patients or family members who are in severe anxiety or panic will be unable to learn from their experience or to learn what you have to teach them until their anxiety level has been reduced. You can be most helpful to patients by helping to channel emotional energy from anxiety into learning.

YOUR REACTIONS TO ANXIETY

You, too, use the coping mechanisms of attack, withdrawal, somatization, and learning when confronted with the vague, unexplained discomfort called anxiety. Anxiety can have a highly disruptive effect on your relationships with patients or clients. An assignment that seemed superficially easy can turn into a draining experience if you or the patient is highly anxious. Patients who are threatened by you or who are worried about their condition can increase your level of anxiety by telegraphing their anxious feelings to you. Since anxiety is an interpersonal experience, obvious anxiety in the other person can often increase anxiety in you. In such situations, you may feel perfectly calm when entering a treatment situation, and then almost immediately begin to feel anxious and uncomfortable. Most often, though, you probably keep your anxiety in check by using a number of coping devices.

Through discussions with community health nurses, it became clear to this author that the source of much of their anxiety was when a patient or doctor did not recognize their authority or did not act in a way they expected him or her to act. For some reason, nurses are especially apt to bristle when a patient or doctor challenges their authority. Perhaps this is because nurses are struggling to prove themselves and to be accepted as equals by other health care professionals. Regardless of the reason why, you may find yourself chiding, scolding, or feeling angry with a patient who challenges your authority. Perhaps this occurs because you are trying to establish yourself as a legitimate authority on the subject of health. However, scolding the patient is not helpful for a number of reasons. First, whenever one person scolds another, the relationship immediately takes on the aspect of a parent-child relationship; when you assume the role of parent, the patient is often coerced into playing the role of (naughty) child. The child role is usually the last role the client should play. This role is one of dependency, helplessness, and inability to problem-solve. Scolding the patient is not helpful to you because other patients who challenge your authority will continue to do so. It is only when you begin to feel secure in yourself and in your usefulness to the patient or client that you will become aware of the fact that it is the patient's challenge that has lead to your feelings of anxiety. Once you are so aware, you will be in a good position to deal more effectively with those patients who challenge your authority.

Challenging the patient's ideas is another way you as nurse attack when threatened. Patients often have good ideas about their care or about what goals they hope to achieve in collaboration with you. Perhaps it is due in part to our nursing education that we feel we must be the authority on all health matters, and that makes it difficult for many nurses to accept and use the patient's ideas. Some comments that could be viewed by clients as an attack on their ideas are: "Of course you don't want to die" or "The doctor and I know this medicine is best for you."

You can avoid experiencing your own anxious feelings by withdrawing from the situation. Calling in sick when assigned a heavy or unreasonable caseload can be a way of withdrawing from an anxiety-producing situation, and of avoiding having to assert yourself with whoever gave you the assignment. Asking to have a difficult patient transferred to another nurse's caseload can be a way of withdrawing from examining what it was about the patient that created anxiety in you. Regarding the nurse-patient relationship as one in which the patient or client is the problem is another way of easing your anxieties at the expense of both you and the patient. By refusing to see the nurse-patient relationship as a process of interaction, you can simply shrug off difficulties in the relationship by labelling the patient as a problem or as too demanding. Distance is thus placed between you and the other, and no real, mutually satisfying relationship can develop.

By using somatization, you need never come to grips with your own anxiety. Feeling excessively fatigued while giving a bedbath to a patient who cried and moaned the whole time, or developing a headache after trying to get another patient to walk are examples of using somatization to deal with your anxious feelings. Somatization can allow you to think about how tired you are or about what a splitting headache you have rather than about why such nurse-patient interactions are so uncomfortable. Although symptoms such as fatigue or headache may relieve the discomfort of anxiety, they are an extreme price to pay for not experiencing your feelings.

None of these reactions allows you more than a temporary breather, and they are certainly not helpful to the patient or client. Although your anxiety is temporarily reduced, it will pop up again whenever a similar anxiety-provoking situation occurs. The only way you can have some assurance that the situation will get better is if you begin to examine the source and meaning of your need to attack, withdraw, or develop physical symptoms when working with certain patients or clients.

INTERVENTIONS

Generally, you need to intervene in cases of anxiety whenever you or the patient does not seem to be able to make any progress toward reaching mutually agreed-upon goals. Whenever goals are not met, you can help the patient, family member, or yourself to identify situations that provoke anxiety. The energy that was previously used to attack, withdraw, or develop a physical symptom is then harnessed to help you deal more effectively with upsetting situations. Different nursing interventions are used for mild and moderate anxiety than when severe anxiety or panic occurs.

Mild and Moderate Anxiety Interventions

When you or the patient is in mild or moderate anxiety, the focus of the intervention is on learning. The first step in the learning process is to become aware of feeling uncomfortable. Often, you may be pretty sure that the patient is anxious; however, he or she may not be aware that this is the source of the difficulty. If you are not sure that anxiety is a problem, observe the patient for signs of withdrawal, anger, somatization, restlessness, decreasing eye contact, rapid and shallow breathing, stammering, and so on. When you observe these signs over a period of time, you can say to the patient, "I wonder if you're feeling anxious (nervous, upset, tense) now." By giving the unexplained discomfort a name, you can help the patient to begin to come to grips with the problem. You may have to help the patient become attuned to his discomfort by focusing his attention on the discomfort a number of times before he is ready to acknowledge that anxiety is what he is experiencing.

Since your own anxiety can influence the course of your relationships with patients, it is important for you to try to learn as much about your own anxiety as possible. Just as you help the patient to give anxiety a name, you can begin to call your own unexplained feeling of discomfort anxiety.

Once both you and the client or patient have named your unexplained discomfort, the next step is to find out what the patient usually does to feel better when he or she is anxious. Patients will often answer that they take long walks, eat, get into an argument with their spouses, call in sick, take a vacation, or try to think through the problem. Many people will not even know what they do to relieve their anxiety. By calling attention to the fact that the patient has learned to deal with anxiety in one way, you have cleared the road for a discussion of what other ways might be used to relieve anxious feelings.

Such discussions point out to both nurse and client that it is possible to take a direct hand in changing one's own behavior.

Likewise, when not with patients or clients, you can begin to examine how you relieve your own anxiety. Questions such as the ones listed in Table 2-5 can help you to learn more about your own anxiety and how it might be affecting your relationships with patients, clients, and family members.

The next step in the learning process is to find out what preceded the feeling of anxiety. You can ask, "What happened right before you felt tense?" "What was going on around you just before your headache started?" or "What was going on just before your diarrhea began?" Such questions help the patient to become more observant of his or her reactions to the environment, and especially to other people. In learning about your own anxiety, you can silently ask yourself the same kinds of questions about what preceded your anxious feeling.

The final step in this learning process is to list other situations where you felt anxious (Peplau, 1962). Often there is a common element to these situations. The common element may be fearing the disapproval of others, experiencing an unexpected event, being with a highly anxious person, or thinking that you

Table 2-5   Questions to Ask When Learning about Your Own Anxiety

Assessment	Exploration
Did my anxiety occur when I was in unfamiliar surroundings?	What kind of surroundings were they?
Did my anxiety occur when I was with a peer or supervisor?	What exactly took place?
Did my anxiety occur when something unexpected happened?	What was it?
Did my anxiety occur when a person I consider important disapproved of me?	What happened step by step?
Did my anxiety occur when I tried to perform a nursing procedure?	Do I need more practice with the procedure, or is something else interfering?
Did my anxiety occur when I lost a patient or friend, or when I thought I might lose something that is important to me?	Exactly what is the meaning of this loss to me?
Did my anxiety get converted into anger, withdrawal, or bodily symptoms?	How might I have learned this method? Is it a method my family uses and as such is familiar to me?
What level of anxiety was I at?	
What were the signs of my anxiety?	
What did I do to relieve my anxiety?	Is this my usual method of reducing anxiety? What other methods are available to me?

cannot perform adequately. There may be some people you work with who seem somewhat anxious and who complain of their inability to manage without your complete assistance. Often these people, although they protest otherwise, function quite well if they are left alone to make individual or family decisions. In such cases, you may want to use a little different intervention. You might comment, "You seem anxious, and you tell me you can't manage, but you have been able to manage quite well." Such a statement not only reminds the person of past successes, but also encourages him or her to take independent action to resolve the problem. In doing this, you do not reject the patient, but rather you encourage independent action while providing support for such action.

You can also help anxious parents who are baffled by the responses of their children by telling them that children get anxious too, and may be uncomfortable due to interactions with their peers, or with school or hospital environments. Parents can be told that children also learn to convert their unexplained discomfort into attack, withdrawal, somatization, and learning. You might also suggest that children learn how to deal with their anxiety by watching their parents. Other parents might be struggling with a problem with their child where the child simply will not talk openly about what is bothering him or her. Many children will not talk in this direct way (Clark, 1977), but can be encouraged to talk through a favorite toy, or by telling a story. Gardner (1975) has suggested simple games and storytelling techniques you can use to communicate with children who are not able to express their feelings directly. Green-Epner (1976) has also suggested therapeutic play techniques that can be adapted for use with children who have difficulty expressing their thoughts and feelings.

You may wonder if these nursing interventions are really worth the effort. You may even think that ignorance is bliss, so why bother with coping devices? In some cases you will not interfere. But when it seems that the patient's current coping devices are not helping, and in fact are creating further difficulties in daily living, nursing intervention is appropriate and necessary.

Severe Anxiety and Panic

When severe anxiety or panic is present, the goal of intervention is to reduce anxiety. One of the most useful interventions for a severely anxious or panicked patient is to be with a person who is calm and who can communicate to the patient that he or she wants to help. In such a case, just your physical presence can be very reassuring and a great deal of talk is not really necessary. Patients or family members in these high levels of anxiety should not be burdened with your statements or questions. The patient is probably overstimulated and does not need further sensory input from you.

Since a high level of anxiety has a disorganizing effect, the patient might be disoriented as to the external environment. It is helpful to orient the patient at short intervals and in concise terms. For example, you might say, "I'll stay with you." A few minutes later you might say, "I'm a nurse" or repeat your name, "I'm Andrea Smith." In another couple of minutes, you could say, "I want to help." Remaining present and giving small bits of orienting information to the patient over a period of time can decrease anxiety. Once the patient is less anxious, you can help the patient to learn from the experience by using statements like, "Tell me what happened" or "What are your feelings about what just happened?"

PREPARING FOR ANXIETY-PROVOKING SITUATIONS

There are always going to be situations that provoke anxiety. New and unexpected situations will crop up, or you will understand what leads to anxious feelings but be at a loss to decrease them as they are actually occurring. There are ways you can prepare for these anxiety-provoking situations, and teach clients and patients to prepare for them.

One way to prepare is to make a mental or written summary of what is expected to happen in upcoming situations. Take the situation to its ultimate conclusion, asking, "What is the worst thing that could happen in this case?" Continue to ask that question until an answer occurs to you. When this question is asked, it is often discovered that the anxiety related to the situation is due to a fear of being rejected, laughed at, not being liked, and so on. Once the hidden fear is out in the open it can be examined. For example, if the fear is "I won't be liked," further questions can be asked, such as, "So what if you're not liked by everyone?" "Is it realistic to be liked by everyone?" "Does it mean I'm less of a person because one person doesn't like me?"

Until you and/or the client become familiar with this technique, there will probably be a tendency to resist tracing an anxiety back to its ultimate source. You or the client may think or say, "This is silly" or "I don't know what the ultimate conclusion is." It is best to keep at it, gently encouraging yourself or another to think about it, and the answer will eventually come to you.

Role-playing situations can be devised to locate the ultimate source of anxiety as well as to practice dealing with an upcoming situation before it occurs. For example, if the anxiety-provoking situation is talking with another about a clinical evaluation, a role-playing situation can be planned to practice this interchange. One person can play the role of supervisor or instructor, while the anxious person takes the part of nurse. Prior to playing out the situation, the anxious person can coach the other on exactly how to play out the scene. After the situation has been role-played, the two players can discuss what went wrong and what went right. Then they can switch roles to get a sense of how the other person might feel. Finally, the original roles can be replayed.

By using this method, you or a client can anticipate any problems that might occur in the actual encounter. Also, hearing yourself perform in a potentially anxiety-provoking situation, as well as receiving feedback from another about your performance can help you to feel more confident. The other role player may make suggestions about how to handle the situation that the anxious person never thought of. Also, the other role player can coach the anxious person in how to present him- or herself in a confident way; some comments that could be made to this effect are, "Look me in the eye when you say that" or "Try sounding more sure of yourself when you say that."

You can introduce this technique to clients in the following way: "I have found role playing to be helpful in teaching people to handle upcoming events more effectively. Let's try it and see if it is helpful to you. The way it works is that you tell us what the upcoming situation is, and you can play the other person in the situation. Then you switch roles with your partner and play the other person. It gives you a feel for what the situation might be like, what you could do instead, and how the other person in the situation might be feeling."

Tape recordings can be used in combination with role playing if it seems important for the role players to hear how they sound. Many times people are not aware of how timid, angry, or guilty they sound until they hear their own voices. If recordings are used, it should only be with the clients' permission.

A third skill you or the client can use to decrease anxiety is the relaxation exercise (Fensterheim, 1971; Benson, 1975). Relaxation exercises are used to help people relax their bodies. When anxiety occurs, body musculature becomes more rigid, pulse and respiration may increase, and a general tightening up occurs. Relaxation exercises inform the body that there is nothing to become tense or threatened about. The first step in one relaxation exercise is to pick out a pleasant relaxing scene. The second step is to practice picturing that scene. Next, the person makes a conscious effort to tense up all body muscles and then relax them, letting all the tension out of the body while exhaling. When the body feels completely relaxed, the pleasant scene that has been chosen is brought to mind. After practicing the pleasant scene and muscle relaxation, the learner is ready for the next step. In this step, the upcoming anxiety-provoking situation is brought to mind, as it is expected to occur, in a step-by-step fashion. As soon as the learner begins to feel anxious, he or she is to say, or think, "Bring back the pleasant scene," to tense up all body muscles and then relax them, and to let all tension out of the body while exhaling. When the learner is again relaxed, he or she is to proceed with the next step of what is expected to happen in the upcoming event. Each time an anxious feeling begins, the learner is to stop and think of the pleasant scene until he or she is completely relaxed. Through repeating this process, the learner can eventually proceed through the entire upcoming situation without experiencing anxiety. Such prepractice will decrease the possibility of becoming highly anxious in the real life situation. When using role-playing or relaxation exercises, it is suggested that you obtain guidance, personal experience, and supervision prior to using them with clients. Although these interventions may appear simple on paper, implementing them requires careful planning and evaluation.

Relaxation exercises can also be used by you or the client in actual anxiety-provoking situations. When feeling anxious, the person can say to him- or herself, "Think of the pleasant scene now." At the same time, he or she can take slow, deep breaths and let tension out of the body by exhaling.

SUMMARY

Anxiety is a vague feeling of unexplained discomfort that is learned and developed in relation to other people. Common sources of anxiety are unmet expectations; unfamiliar, unexpected, or embarrassing situations; disapproval from significant other people; and situations that demand a performance that the person thinks he or she is not capable of performing.

Because anxiety is such an uncomfortable feeling, both you and your clients tend to convert this feeling into anger, withdrawal, physical symptoms, or learning. At the mild and moderate anxiety levels, a person is still capable of learning, and can be helped to do so by naming the feeling, by becoming aware of relief behaviors, by figuring out what happened just prior to the feeling of anxiety, and by examining common elements in situations that provoke anxiety. In cases of severe anxiety and panic, learning does not occur. Automatic and repetitive behaviors can be observed. A comforting physical presence, concise, orienting statements, and a decrease in sensory input can help to lower anxiety to a point where learning can occur.

You can learn and teach others to prepare for anxiety-provoking situations in a number of ways: what is the worst thing that could happen exercise, role playing, tape recordings, and relaxation exercises.

PRACTICE EXERCISES

List some situations that create anxiety in you in each of the areas listed below.

1 The unexpected
   a
   b
   c
   What would be the worst unexpected patient situation that you could encounter? Develop this situation in your mind, taking it to its ultimate conclusion. Ask yourself how you might deal with the ultimate conclusion if it should occur.
2 The embarrassing
   a
   b
   c
   What nurse-patient interactions do you find embarrassing? Why do you suppose you get embarrassed? Imagine an embarrassing situation where you do

not get embarrassed. Enjoy the feeling of being calm and comfortable in a situation that has previously caused you embarrassment. The next time you find yourself in a similar situation, try to recapture that calm, comfortable feeling.

3 The unfamiliar
    a
    b
    c
    Try to figure out what aspects of each situation are anxiety-provoking. Is it the physical environment, not knowing the people present, not knowing what the correct thing to do is, or something else?

REVIEW

Definition

Define anxiety.

Listing

1 List four sources of anxiety.

_____

_____

2 List four levels of anxiety.

_____

_____

3 List nursing interventions that are useful for each level of anxiety listed below.
    a mild or moderate anxiety

_____

_____

    b severe anxiety or panic

_____

_____

Matching Terms

Match client coping devices with the examples by placing the correct letter in front of the appropriate coping device.

Coping devices	Examples
1 _____ withdrawal	a tension headache
2 _____ somatization	b "You don't know what you're doing!"
3 _____ anger	c getting diarrhea before an important test
4 _____ learning	d calling in sick
	e feeling tired without having exerted oneself

REFERENCES

Benson, H. 1975. *The relaxation response.* New York: Morrow.

Braden, C. et al. 1976. Encouraging client self-discovery. *American Journal of Nursing* 76, 3:444–446.

Clark, C. 1977. Psychotherapy with the resistant child. *Perspectives in Psychiatric Care* 15, 3:122–125.

Fensterheim, H. 1971. *Help without psychoanalysis.* New York: Stein and Day.

Finch, A. et al. 1975. Effects of two types of failure on anxiety. *Journal of Abnormal Psychology* 84, 5(October):583–585.

Gardner, R. 1975. *Psychotherapeutic approaches to the resistant child.* New York: Aronson.

Green-Epner, C. 1976. The dying child. In *The dying patient: a supportive approach*, ed. R. Caughill, pp. 125–154. Boston: Little, Brown.

Himle, D. et al. 1975. Behavioral indices of anxiety and locus of control. *Psychological Reprints* 37, 3(December):1008.

Peplau, H. 1952. Unexplained discomfort. In *Interpersonal relations in nursing*, pp. 119–187. New York: Putnam.

_____ 1962. Interpersonal techniques: the crux of psychiatric nursing. *American Journal of Nursing* 62, 6(June):50–54.

_____ 1963. A working definition of anxiety. In *Some clinical approaches to psychiatric nursing*, eds. S. Burd and M. Marshall, pp. 323–327. New York: Macmillan.

Petrillo, M., and Sarger, S. 1972. *Emotional care of hospitalized children.* Philadelphia: Lippincott.

Prytula, R. et al. 1975. Analysis of general anxiety scale for children and draw-a-person measure of general anxiety level in elementary school children. *Perceptual Motor Skills* 41, 3(December):995–1007.

Snaith, R. et al. 1976. The Leeds scale for self-assessment of anxiety and depression. *British Journal of Psychiatry* 128(February):156–165.

Stephens, K. 1973. A toddler's separation anxiety. *American Journal of Nursing* 73, 9:1553–1555.

Sullivan, H. 1953. *The interpersonal theory of psychiatry.* New York: Norton.

Tubbs, A. 1970. Nursing intervention to shorten anxiety-ridden transition periods. *Nursing Outlook* 18(July):27.

Chapter 3

Conflict, Guilt, and Responsibility

LEARNING OBJECTIVES

When you finish this chapter, you should be able to:

- Identify situations where conflict is operating
- Identify situations where irrational guilt is occurring
- State a reasonable definition of health care responsibility

Issues of conflict and guilt are often related to and influenced by how you and the client define degrees of responsibility. Because nurses are apt to become embroiled in these issues, it is important for you to think about their meaning and to be able to assess and intervene in situations of conflict and guilt.

CONFLICT

Conflict is a concept that has relevance for both you and your clients. Conflict occurs whenever you or your client(s) have opposing goals; it also occurs when the needs of an individual are in opposition to each other or oppose the needs of others. Most of us learn and adhere to a number of values that are difficult to reconcile. For example, as nurse you have probably been taught to meet all your patient's needs, while at the same time you are also supposed to encourage his or her independence. In addition, you have probably learned that you must complete your task assignment in an efficient way and keep objective records (i.e., please the boss or instructor), yet you must also cater to the client and offer warmth and concern (i.e., please the client via mothering, humanistic, and technical skills). On top of meeting these somewhat opposing goals, you must also reconcile your own physiological, safety, interpersonal, and self-actualizing needs (Maslow, 1970) with those of your client.

So, as far as you are concerned, you have several sets of opposing goals to reconcile. Therefore, you will probably be faced with some of the following questions that can create conflict:

How do I assist family members while at the same time helping them to maintain their independence?

How do I please the supervisor (instructor) and still please the family?

How do I support the identified patient* when other family members make demands on me or complain about my care?

How do I decide if plans for care are realistic or if the family is just not ready to change?

How can I continue to see a family when I know unsafe or unhealthy practices continue to occur despite my teaching attempts?

How can I continue to feel good about my work when my clients do not improve or appreciate my efforts?

Families with whom you work will probably also have opposing sets of goals including some of the following:

How can we please the nurse yet satisfy ourselves?

How can I (the identified patient) get better without making too many new demands on the family?

How can I (the identified patient) get better yet still get my needs to be taken care of met?

How can we obtain health care without giving up our independence and opinions?

As a nurse, you have a number of tasks to complete in order to deal effectively with conflict in yourself and in others. One task is to learn some signs that indicate conflict is occurring. Because goals are in opposition when

---

*The identified patient, or IP, is the first family member to acknowledge his or her need for help and to enter the health care system.

conflict is present there is a tendency to move toward and then away from goals (vacillation), to have difficulty making decisions (indecisiveness), and to begin to and then to abruptly stop communicating (blocking).

Bearing in mind the above examples of conflicts that may occur in the course of administering nursing care, consider the following signs that could indicate that conflict is occurring in you:

Alternating doing things for family members with chiding them to take responsibility for their actions

Taking more than the usual amount of time with a family and then rushing to write up your report and leaving work late

Trying to work with the IP but being distracted by your desire to help and/or your need to fend off family members at the same time

Writing and rewriting nursing care plans but deciding not to share them with the family

Teaching families healthy behaviors and then being ambivalent about continuing to see them when they do not follow through on your advice

Alternating your work with families with actions to end the relationship when their improvement or their appreciation of your efforts is not forthcoming

Bearing in mind the above examples of conflicts that may occur in the nurse-family relationship, consider the following signs that conflict is occurring within a family:

The family alternates between doing what the nurse suggests and doing what family members want or feel comfortable with.

The IP alternates between acting independently and asking family members or you to take care of him or her.

The members of the family alternate between agreeing to do what you suggest and carrying out their own ideas.

Once you have identified the opposing pulls you or the family is experiencing, your next task is to accept the idea that both aspects of a conflict situation are initially not known to the people involved in the conflict. Although it may seem obvious to you what is the correct action or decision for family members to take, these conclusions are probably not obvious to them. At times you may feel frustrated or as though you are running around in circles trying to please the client, the family, and/or a supervisor or instructor. Although you may experience increased tension and stress, you may not be aware that the source of these feelings is conflict. You can use the assessment questions in Table 3-1 to help you determine whether you or family members are in conflict.

Table 3-1 Conflict Assessment Questions

Questions about the nurse	Questions about family members
Do I alternate between making decisions for family members and chiding them for not making their own decisions?	Do family members agree to comply with your suggestions and then do the opposite?
Do I alternate between doing things *for* the IP or family members and expecting them to be independent?	Do family members seem to have difficulty making health care decisions?
Do I feel unable to set limits on and priorities for the care that I give to the family and for my own performance?	Does the IP alternate between acting independently and trying to get you or family members to do things for him or her?
Do I feel unable to balance my time between work with family members and administrative demands?	Does the IP agree that he or she should change, but never seems to be able to change?

Once you assess conflict in yourself, you can use Table 3-2 to help you to resolve your conflict. You might use the same method with clients, but remember that it is first necessary to help them to become aware that conflict is occurring. Initially, you can serve as an active listener and sounding board. Sometimes being listened to helps people in conflict to resolve their dilemma. At other times, more active interventions may be needed.

If the conflict seems to be in the area of decision making, you might comment, "Making decisions is a difficult task; perhaps I can help you to examine the pros and cons of both sides of the issue." If the conflict seems to be related

Table 3-2 Decision or Behavior: Setting Priorities for Care

Directions for the Exercise

1 Take a piece of paper and divide it into two columns.
2 In the left column write down the reasons why you choose a decision or behavior.
3 In the right column write down the reasons why the decision or behavior is not a good idea, or what factors might mitigate against it.
4 Decide if the pros outweigh the cons or vice versa.
5 If you are unable to decide alone, talk your ideas over with an objective person whom you trust.

Pros or advantages	Cons or inhibiting factors
1 I would be less easily manipulated by clients.	1 I may have to admit to my own needs.
2 I could use my time more efficiently.	2 It is not always easy to set priorities.
3 I would feel more satisfied that I had accomplished my goals.	3 I may have to acknowledge that I have limitations as well as strengths.

to the client's seeming willingness to comply with your advice, you might comment, "You seem to agree with what I suggest, but something seems to be preventing you from carrying it out. Perhaps together we can figure out what that might be." If the conflict seems to be centered around the IP's inability to act independently and in a consistent manner, you might decide not to discuss the conflict at all, but rather to praise any movements toward independence, and ignore and not comment on his or her dependent actions.

GUILT

People feel guilty when they perceive that their abilities are not sufficient to fulfill the demands of a given situation. Guilt occurs when you or the client feel inadequate, or that you have made an error in judgment or have committed an inappropriate action. Because guilt is an uncomfortable feeling, we tend to try to remedy the situation through self-punishment or self-recrimination.

Guilt can be seen as a carry-over from childhood when parental approval was sought, and disapproval was forthcoming (Peplau, 1952). Most often, guilt operates outside of our awareness, but it can be observed in our actions. Some cues that guilt is occurring in a person are asking to be hurt or verbally punished, asking that services or rewards be withheld, and setting up goals that are impossible to attain and that are unrewarding.

For growth to occur, the guilt feeling must be recognized and realistic expectations for the situation must be explored. For many nurses, guilt is caused by saying "no" to clients or authority figures. Many people, but particularly women, seem to have difficulty setting limits on other people's behavior. Part of this difficulty seems to be tied to cultural learnings about women being assertive (Grissum, 1976). Taubman (1976) has categorized the fears that underlie guilt about being assertive. These include fear of not being liked, fear of rejection, fear of retaliation, fear of loss of control, fear of learning the truth about oneself. In nursing, assertiveness amounts to setting goals, acting on these goals in a clear and consistent way, and taking responsibility for the consequences of our actions.

Learning what it is in you that prohibits assertive behavior and evokes guilt is part of dealing with irrational guilt. Once you know what lies behind your feelings of guilt, it will be easier for you to make a realistic assessment of your difficulties in this area and to find a workable solution. Table 3-3 lists some questions that you can ask yourself in order to assess your tendency to feel guilty; if you answer "yes" to all or most of the questions, it is important for you to work toward a resolution in this area since your feelings are bound to influence your ability to work successfully with clients. When you shy away from asserting your rights as a person and as a nurse, your resentment and anger will go underground and then emerge in the form of snide remarks, punitive tactics, blame of others, and attempts to make others feel guilty.

Table 3-3 Assessing Guilt Potential

Questions for the nurse	Questions for the client
Do I have difficulty saying "no" when a client, supervisor, or instructor makes an unrealistic demand on me?	Does the client have difficulty saying "no" to others?
Do I change my goals for a family based on what seems to be an impulsive whim on its part?	Does the client change his or her direction merely to please others?
Do I work overtime even though I have an important engagement or class?	Does the client offer to spend time with others at the expense of his or her own needs?
Do I seem to try too hard to please the client, supervisor, or instructor?	Does the client seem to be trying to please me rather than to meet his or her health goals?
Do I overapologize when I'm late or when I wish to leave early?	Does the client overapologize?
Do I feel guilty if I take a few extra minutes for lunch occasionally?	Does the client offer excuses for every action that is self-initiated?
Do I get upset when someone points out a mistake I've made?	Does the client get upset when his or her limitations are discussed?
Do I withdraw from others without explanation?	Does the client withdraw from others without explanation?
Do I fear failing or getting fired?	Does the client mention his or her fears of failing?
Do I have a hard time telling clients and people I work with when I feel angry or upset?	Does the client have extreme difficulty telling you or others that he or she is angry or upset?
Do I feel guilty when people say, "How can you do this to me?" "If you cared about me, you would . . ." or "You are really disappointing me . . ." etc.	Does the client comply without question when told what to do or when asked to complete an action?
Do I have difficulty stating what I want from others?	Can the client tell you and others what he or she wants or expects?
Do I expect that things will turn out all right if I just wait things out?	Does the client sit back passively without actively trying to meet his or her goals?
Do I expect peers, clients, or supervisors to know what I want without telling them?	Does the client seem to expect others to read her or his mind and to know what is needed or wanted?
Do I call in sick and then worry about it?	Does the client miss appointments and then report worrying about having missed them?
Do I fear being disliked?	Does the client indicate fear of the disapproval of others?

When working with clients who show signs of guilt, you can help them to identify the feeling by asking them a question such as, "What do you feel in a situation like the one you just described?" It is always helpful to phrase a question to determine the client's feeling, rather than to assume the feeling being experienced is guilt. First, you might ask the client to identify the feeling. If the client is unable to do so and if you have noticed that the client consistently exhibits one or more of the behaviors listed in Table 3-3, you might make a comment such as, "I've noticed that you seem to have a hard time asking me for help. I wonder if you feel guilty about doing so, even though that's why I'm here." The client may then be able to say, "Yes, I don't want to bother you, but I guess you are here to help me," or something to that effect. Once clients are aware of their guilty feeling, it will become possible for you to discuss with them whether they think it is reasonable to expect everyone to like them or to demand excuses for their behavior. If the client's guilt is deep-seated, you may decide to refer him or her to a nurse psychotherapist or mental health counselor who would be able to focus more intensively on this issue. Clients who have deep-seated guilt will usually not be able to identify their guilt so readily and are often preoccupied with feelings of their own worthlessness. Their inability to identify their guilt feelings as well as their continued preoccupation with being unworthy of your help can lead to a block in the nurse-client relationship. If you find that the block persists, you may choose to refer the client for more intensive counseling.

RESPONSIBILITY

Conflict and guilt influence expectations for responsibility. Nurses or clients who are in conflict about how to perform, and who base their criteria for effective nursing care only on client approval are most apt to assume greater responsibility for the nurse-client relationship than is reasonable.

A rule of thumb for you to remember is that you are responsible for structuring health care practices and discussions while you are with the client, but that you cannot be responsible for his behavior when you are not with him. A corollary of this is that although you can take responsibility for structuring the direction of care while with a client, there is no way you can force him to think or feel in a particular way. You are even restricted as to how much control you have over clients' actions, since, unless you physically force them to submit, you cannot take responsibility for their actions.

As a group, nurses are overly responsible people and therefore need to guard against taking over and doing *for* others. Toman (1976) has found that first-born children with younger siblings learn to take the lead in caring for others. If you have had this kind of family experience, you need to be especially on guard against your tendencies to be overly responsible. As a community health nurse, you will work with clients who are ambulatory or who are functioning in the community on some level. Working in the home underlines the fact that families are primarily responsible for their own behavior, since they have not given over control of their environment to an institution. Even clinic patients retain more responsibility for their lives than do hospitalized or institutionalized people.

Since other people besides nurses have trouble sorting out which responsibilities are realistic and which are not, it is not unusual that you will come in contact with families that may try to engage you to hospitalize or institutionalize what the family considers to be the sick, bad, or weak part of itself. By turning over this decision to you, the family abrogates its responsibility for its own functioning. As a nurse, you may be asked to decide when a family member should be hospitalized or placed in a nursing home or in some other type of institution. By refusing to make this decision, you can help the family to move to a higher level of functioning. This is not to suggest that you should avoid the decision. Rather, it is suggested that you tell the family that you will help it to examine the pros and cons of the decision and that you will provide information and guidance so that it can make an effective decision. Table 3-4 lists steps that you may take to help guide the family toward making an effective decision.

Of course, there may be emergencies or acute illnesses where action is preferable to discussion. However, hospitalizations and institutionalizations usually do not stem from such extreme situations. If you know you have difficulty restraining yourself from doing something *to* or *for* a client, it will be useful for you to examine whether you decide health care issues because you feel

Table 3-4 Guiding Effective Family Decisions

Steps	Examples of nursing actions
1 State the problem clearly	"We're here to talk about the pros and cons of Mrs. T going to a nursing home."
2 Elaborate parts of the problem	"Perhaps each person could tell how Mrs. T's going to a nursing home would affect the family."
3 Encourage family to develop alternate solutions	"What alternatives are there right now?"
4 Keep discussion relevant to the decision at hand	"I think we're off the point; let's get back to . . ."
5 Summarize frequently	"So far we've talked about the disadvantages, but not the advantages."
6 Encourage family to test out solutions	"How about a visit to the nursing home by the family, including Mrs. T, to see what it's like?"
7 Test for consensus	"What is everyone's reaction to the idea?"
8 Decision is reached	"I guess you all agree, even Mrs. T, that the nursing home is the best solution for right now."

comfortable doing so or because the client is unable to do for himself. You may be surprised to see how well families can function with minimal information, support, and direction from you. Gresham (1976) has noted that helpgivers are apt to treat the elderly as less capable than they are. It may also be that help-givers are apt to treat many clients as less capable than they are.

If you are unsure of your performance and need approval from others, you are probably more likely to overprotect or underprotect clients. In addition to the individual differences operating to decrease nurses' assertiveness and to increase their feelings of conflict and guilt, there are group and work setting factors that influence community nursing practice.

A major influence is the independent and isolated practice of some com-munity health settings. In hospitals, institutions, and clinics, staff members are often in constant contact with one another. Because you may be working pri-marily with clients, you may receive little peer and administrative support. This may lead to your subjectifying and overidentifying with family members. Because this is likely to occur, it will be useful for you to participate in (or sug-gest the formation of) peer review and peer support groups.

By meeting together with other community health nurses, you can provide support for each other by sharing common reactions to the dynamics of specific family situations and of community health nursing situations. Some common reactions that community health nurses seem to deal with better as a result of peer group support include: performance anxiety, conflict, guilt, and responsi-bility for health care; helplessness and anger when dealing with depressed people or those who have chronic illnesses; feelings of aggressiveness and/or avoidance when dealing with doctors or supervisors.

A peer review group is another source of input and objectivity that you can use to support and evaluate your nursing practice. Some activities of nurse peer review groups are: writing sets of health/wellness outcome criteria, comparing nursing care results with outcome criteria, identifying possible causes for not meeting criteria, and recommending and reporting ways to improve outcomes (Zimmer, 1974).

SUMMARY

Conflict occurs whenever you or your clients have opposing goals. Guilt occurs when you or the client feels inadequate, that an error in judgment has been made, or that an inappropriate action has been taken. Conflict and guilt influ-ence expectations for responsibility. If you are conflicted over how to perform your task and over whether to base your performance criteria on the client's approval, you are apt to assume greater responsibility for the nurse-client rela-tionship than is reasonable. Assessments and interventions for conflict and guilt both in yourself and in your clients can lead to more realistic expectations regarding who is responsible for what in the relationship.

PRACTICE EXERCISES

1 Using Table 3-1, choose several families and evaluate their level of conflict.
2 Use Table 3-1 to evaluate your own level of conflict.
3 Use Table 3-2 to begin to resolve your own or a client's opposing goals.
4 Use Table 3-3 to evaluate your level of guilt; a "yes" answer to most of the questions indicates that there is a high potential for guilt to interfere with effective nursing care. Decide how you will resolve these feelings so as to be more effective in your practice.

REVIEW

Multiple-choice Questions

1 Identify the situation(s) below where conflict may be operating.
   a One day you take complete care of the patient and the next day you ask him to assume complete care of himself.
   b You keep changing health care goals despite the fact that the family is experiencing no real change in its growth.
   c You overapologize for taking a few minutes off from work once in a while.
   d One day the family decides to send a member to a nursing home and the next day it decides to keep the member at home.
2 Identify the situation(s) below where irrational guilt seems to be operating.
   a The IP agrees to try out a new procedure, but then never does.
   b You have difficulty saying "no" to others.
   c One day the IP does a self-care procedure beautifully and the next day he or she, in tears, asks for your assistance.
   d You call in sick and then spend the whole day worrying about what your supervisor or instructor will say when you return to work.

Definition

Define in reasonable terms what constitutes your responsibility as a health care giver.

REFERENCES

Bradford, L. et al. 1976. How to diagnose group problems. In *Management for nurses*, eds. S. Stone et al., pp. 133–146. St. Louis: Mosby.

Fagin, C. 1975. Nurses' rights. *American Journal of Nursing* 75, 1:82–85.

Fensterheim, H., and Baer, J. 1975. *Don't say "yes" when you want to say "no."* New York: Dell.

Gresham, M. 1976. The infantilization of the elderly: a developing concept. *Nursing Forum* 15:195–210.

Grissum, M., and Spengler, C. 1976. *Womanpower and health care.* Boston: Little, Brown.

Johnson, K., and Zimmerman, M. 1975. Peer review in a health department. *American Journal of Nursing* 75, 4:618–619.

Maslow, A. H. 1970. *Motivation and personality.* 2d ed. New York: Harper and Row.

Nassau, J. 1975. *Choosing a nursing home.* New York: Funk and Wagnalls.

Nisbett, R., and Valins, S. 1971. *Perceiving causes of one's own behavior.* Morristown, N.J.: General Learning Press.

Peplau, H. 1952. *Interpersonal relations in nursing.* New York: Putnam.

Plachy, R. 1976. Delegation and decision-making. In *Management for nurses,* eds. S. Stone et al., pp. 58–69. St. Louis: Mosby.

Smith, M. 1975. *When I say no, I feel guilty.* New York: Dial.

Taubman, G. 1976. *How to become an assertive woman.* New York: Pocket.

Thomstad, B. et al. 1975. Changing the rules of the doctor-nurse game. *Nursing Outlook* 23, 7:422–427.

Toman, W. 1976. *Family Constellation.* 3d ed. New York: Springer.

Wilfong, M. et al. 1976. Starting a system for evaluating quality of care: process and product. *Maternal Child Nursing* 1:141–144.

Wrightsman, L. 1972. *Social psychology for the seventies.* Monterey, Calif.: Brooks/Cole.

Zimmer, M. 1974. Quality assurance for outcomes of patient care. *Nursing Clinics of North America* 9, 2:305–315.

Chapter 4

Grief, Depression,
and Violent Behavior

LEARNING OBJECTIVES

When you finish this chapter, you should be able to:

- Identify interventions for stages of the grief process
- State four interventions for learned helplessness
- Identify indicants of high suicide potential
- List three interventions for a person who expresses suicidal thoughts
- Identify indicants of potential child abuse

At first glance it may seem curious to find grief, depression, and violence in the same chapter. However, depression can be viewed as the result of unsuccessful grieving and can be explained as frustration or hostility turned inward. Violent actions such as suicide, homicide, or child abuse frequently are also the result of frustration and hostility. Perhaps the unifying thread among these behaviors is anger: in grief, anger is expressed and is potentially resolved; in depression, anger is turned inward and is not resolved; in suicide, anger is turned against oneself instead of being used as an energy source for dealing with one's life situation; in homicide, some cases of which are actually suicides where one person provokes another to kill him or her, anger is used as an energy source, but is directed in an antisocial way; in child abuse, parents who themselves were abused act out their own frustration and anger by harming their children.

GRIEF

Grief can be viewed as the expected response to a loss. It is the series of internal reactions that people have when they lose a loved one, a body part or function, a mental or physical capacity, or a comfortable environment. Every growth experience or change results in a loss and a need to grieve that loss. Losses can be expected, e.g., those that occur in the course of normal growth and developmental processes, or they can be unexpected, e.g., accidents.

The more the person has invested emotionally in an object, situation, or relationship, the stronger that person's reaction will be to the loss. Since emotional attachments cannot be measured accurately, you cannot assume that the loss of a finger or a pet is of less or more importance than the loss of speech, sexual ability, or a family member.

You can assume, however, that people who do not respond to their losses tend to have recurring difficulty in resolving loss, adapting to change, and proceeding through growth and development periods. For example, mothers who were separated emotionally or physically from their own parents and who never resolved this separation will have difficulty managing their own children.

Grief is a helpful, although painful, process that helps people to cope with overwhelming events in a gradual way. People who never learn to grieve or who fear strong feelings may have difficulty reestablishing homeostasis, and may misinterpret or try to repress their grief. It is not uncommon for people to seek psychiatric help because they misinterpret the sadness that they are feeling or because they are unable to complete the grief process and are depressed as a result.

Grief can be thought of as a series of steps; however, in practice, people rarely progress in an orderly way from one step to the next. The first reaction to a loss is shock or disbelief; high levels of anxiety correspond to this stage.

Once reality sinks in, there is a stage of denial where the person may act as if the loss had not occurred. Comments you might hear are: "I'm not dying" (or refusal of a dying person to mention death); "You should have helped more" (a displacement and projection of one's own feelings of anger or impotence); "I'll just get up and walk" (after a bilateral leg amputation). Behaviors that could exemplify denial include: not responding when others call you by a recently acquired name or title; driving when intoxicated; smoking after lung surgery.

Denial frequently comes and goes throughout the process of resolving a loss, and may overlap with the next stage, anger. In this stage, people begin to realize that they are really angry about the loss and they begin to be preoccupied with the loss. "Why did this have to happen now?" or "Why me?" are comments heard from people at this point in their grief. Behaviors such as provoking arguments with others, blaming you, blaming family members "for the mess I'm in" are also indicators of the anger stage.

If the grieving person can move through the stages of anger and denial, he or she will eventually accept and/or successfully adapt to the change. The grief process proceeds in essentially the same manner whether the client, family, or you are grieving a developmental or situational loss, including the death of a loved one. For this reason, you need to have a working knowledge of the grief process, of how you react to various behaviors that are typical of the grief process, of what signs indicate that grieving is not taking place, and of how you can assist people to grieve successfully. Table 4-1 lists some experiences that may cause grief and details the indicants and stages of the grief process.

Your reactions will often parallel the client's or family's reactions. Thus, your feelings and reactions can be useful barometers of how the family is dealing with its losses. Questions you can ask to assess your reactions when dealing with families that are suffering losses are listed in Figure 4-1.

There are a number of signs that you can use to assess a person's or family's failure to grieve (see Figure 4-2). No one sign is necessarily indicative of real difficulty, but if family members show several or all of these signs, it is important to refer them for intensive counseling or psychotherapy.

Interventions for grief vary depending on the stage of the grieving process. In the shock/disbelief stage, it is most useful to the client for you to remain present and to decrease his or her sensory input. Since this is a time of high anxiety, interventions that are useful for severe anxiety will be useful now (see Chapter 2, "Anxiety").

In the denial stage, it is important that you allow the denial to be expressed, but that you show interest and concern for the person as a person. It can be helpful to both you and the client for you to sit silently with him or her, noting nonverbal signals of isolation and loneliness, and making comments such as, "You may not feel like talking right now, but I'll sit with you a while" or "When you're ready to talk, I'm ready to listen."

In the anger stage, it is important that you make yourself available to the person despite his or her angry statements. You need to be aware of any tendency that you might have to withdraw when you are confronted with the anger of another. You can reflect angry comments and even encourage them by saying, "You're angry and it's OK to talk about it with me."

In all of these stages, you can expect very little ability on the part of your clients to learn new procedures or to assume full control of their bodies and lives. It is only in the acceptance stage when people have completed most of their grieving that they are ready and able to learn. Some people may pass through their grief process relatively quickly and be ready and open to your

Table 4-1 Some Losses Where Grief Can Be Expected

Experience	Possible indicants of grief	Grief stage
Tooth extraction	Child cries	Shock, disbelief
	"Mommy, bad!"	Anger
	"Where is the tooth?"	Preoccupation with loss
	"I'll put it under my pillow"	Acceptance
Entering school	Child cries	Shock, disbelief, anger
	Refuses to go to school	Denial, anger
	Goes to school	Acceptance, wish to please
Unwanted pregnancy	Crying	Shock, disbelief, anger
	"It won't change anything."	Denial
	"Why didn't you get a vasectomy (tubal ligation)?"	Anger
	"I guess we'll be OK."	Acceptance
Promotion	"I don't deserve this!"	Disbelief
	Refuses to answer to new title	Denial
	"This job is a real pain!"	Anger
	Assumes new title and responsibilities	Acceptance
Middle age	"What? 50 new grey hairs!"	Shock, disbelief, anger
	"I'm really still young."	Denial
	Frantic attempts to prove youth via dress, work, or sexual activity	Denial
	"How can *I* be getting older?"	Anger
	Reorders life goals	Acceptance
Mastectomy	"Oh, no!"	Shock, disbelief
	Acts as if surgery had not occurred	Denial
	"Why me?"	Anger
	Resumes active social life	Acceptance

teaching efforts. Others seem to become stuck in one stage and remain there for some time; some people never move past the denial stage. Others may never reach the acceptance stage because they get sidetracked by depression.

DEPRESSION

There are a number of different explanations for *depression*. One is that it is the result of frustration and hostility being turned inward. In this sense, depression differs from an expected grief reaction. In a grief reaction, anger is not turned inward and one's self-esteem remains reasonably high; there is a sense

Figure 4-1 Questions to Ask to Assess Your Responses to Grief in Yourself and in Your Clients

Do my reactions parallel those of the family, for example:
  Do I feel highly anxious and disorganized?
    (Shock/disbelief stage)

  Do I overemphasize task and procedures so I won't have to focus on the loss?
    (Denial stage)

  Do I act as if there has been no loss?
    (Denial stage)

  Do I feel angry when a grieving family member shows anger?
    (Anger stage)

  Do I feel comfortable dealing with the loss of a family member?
    (Acceptance stage)

of emptiness, but the emptiness is perceived as being outside of oneself and in the environment. In depression, self-esteem is low (or lowered) and the emptiness is perceived as being inside of oneself.

Everyone has minor depressive episodes with symptoms such as insomnia, lack of appetite, thoughts of not doing well or of never succeeding or that life does not seem worth living, fatigue, and inability to take an interest in what is happening in the world. Usually these periods pass, and are replaced with a renewed and vigorous interest in life and living.

For some people, depression becomes a vicious cycle where, as they feel more and more unworthy, they withdraw, become preoccupied with their body functions, and feel more worthless and depressed. This is probably because people need to experience satisfaction over how they relate to others and over how they master their environment. Therefore, being preoccupied with minor aches

Figure 4-2 Signs of Failure to Grieve Successfully

No reaction at the time of the loss

Physical or emotional symptoms that continue to occur more than 1 year after the loss

Increased anxiety at the approach of the anniversary of the loss

Persistent feelings of guilt

Decreased sense of self-esteem

Withdrawal from family and friends for more than 1 year after the loss

Increase of physical symptoms with no organic basis that seem to be related to the loss

Inability to discuss the loss in a calm manner more than 1 year after the loss and pains and with guilt about past experiences drives other people away and leaves little time for establishing relationships with others and for mastering the environment. Figure 4-3 illustrates this vicious cycle of depression. People who tend to retreat into depression may view conflict as bad rather than as a necessary component in a growth process. Women especially seem to be struggling with this issue more and more, perhaps as a result of the Women's Movement. Many factors, including their own ambivalent feelings about being assertive and about being themselves, have combined to lead to a recent increase in depression among women (Miller, 1976).

A relatively new framework for regarding depression is the *learned helplessness model* (Hooker, 1976), which offers the view that the person thinks he or she has no influence on the outcome of events and so he or she does not even try to influence the environment. Seligman (1975) explains a *reactive depression* (reaction to a specific loss) as the real or imagined loss of control over life events and the belief in one's helplessness. Minuchin and others (1975) expand on a variation of the learned helplessness model by showing how families reinforce what seems to be helpless or hopeless behavior but what is essentially an attempt to control others. For example, Minuchin views the behavior of some children with difficulties such as diabetes, asthma, and *anorexia nervosa* as a way to control others and to be controlled by them. One of his interventions with families where these illness processes occur is to relabel the child's behavior from "You are sick" to "You are controlling the whole family by having these crises."

If one considers the idea that people develop styles of relating to others, interpersonal learning takes on a great importance. Some people may learn to act helpless as a way of coping because they believe that they have no control over events, when in fact they actually do or can affect events. This learning may have occurred because they have been unable to resolve crises effectively (Hooker, 1976).

This view has implications for you in your work to help people resolve their grief successfully. If people fail repeatedly, if they are unable to resolve separations and losses effectively, or if they feel that they have no effect on outcomes, they may assume learned helplessness as a way of coping with life situations.

Learned helplessness also has implications for you in your work with people who have already adopted this way of seeing themselves and of relating to other people. Some interventions that you can use include introducing structured

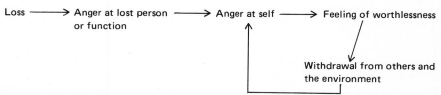

Figure 4-3 Depression as a vicious cycle.

tasks, utilizing role-playing situations, using firmness to evoke anger and praising its expression, and assessing your own need to have the client(s) like you.

Structured Tasks

If you accept as a framework that people with learned helplessness styles have a self-concept of not being able to do anything right, that they attach a negative value to failure, criticism, and expression of feeling, and that they believe that they are always in the wrong, you can structure experiences to counteract previous learning experiences. One way to do this is to start with very simple, specific tasks where success is assured. It is also important to praise the person when the goal is attained, and not to respond when people fail or when they start to berate themselves. For example, a long-range goal for a very depressed person may be to interact with others in a social situation. Expecting a highly depressed person to move from complete withdrawal to spontaneous interaction with others is unrealistic. Rather, shape that person's behaviors and move him or her toward that goal. An early step that you might take in this direction is to have the person move out of his or her bedroom and walk with you to the living room. On the next visit, the goal may be for the client to walk to the kitchen, or to sit outside the house with you. Determining the progression of events that are needed to achieve the long-range goal is time-consuming, but such a plan has a greater chance of succeeding than does merely telling the client, "You need to get out and socialize with others." Table 4-2 presents a chart that one community health nurse used to structure her work with a depressed client. The chart was posted in the client's home; progress toward the goal was visible and served to further reinforce movement toward it. The kind of steps that are taken toward the goal and their magnitude may be adjusted depending on the degree of debility of the client. For homebound or bedbound people, very small steps such as turning to face the nurse or assisting in the process of combing one's own hair may be beginning or middle steps away from learned helplessness.

Table 4-2   A Structured Task Chart for a Depressed Client

Activity	Date accomplished
Knock on neighbor's door alone, go in, and visit for 5 minutes	11/20
Knock on neighbor's door alone	11/4
Knock on neighbor's door, go in with nurse, and visit for 5 minutes	10/25
Walk to neighbor's house with nurse	10/17
Walk 1 block with nurse	10/14
Walk down driveway	10/8
Sit outside for 15 minutes with nurse	10/6
Walk to kitchen	10/3
Walk to living room from bedroom	10/1

Role-Playing Situations

What prevents many people from attempting action is their fear that they will fail. By devising role-playing situations you can help a client to play out and run through his or her worst fears. For example, suppose a client with multiple sclerosis who is in a wheelchair never goes to social outings because she knows that she will be too uncomfortable. In such a case, it can be helpful to say, "All right, let's pretend you are at the outing; now what do you think would happen first?" You can then begin to understand what leads to the client's discomfort in social situations. Many times it is the fear that others will deny her existence or be too overprotective and try to do everything for her. If the first fear surfaces, you can say, "OK, I'll act like I don't even know you're here, and you do what you want." After one play through it may be clear to both you and the client that she can move or talk in certain ways to better assure that others will pay attention to her. These better ways can also be role-played. Once a person has some experience in actually saying the words, and in considering the pros and cons of one or another way to deal with a situation, she will often replace her fear of the unknown with a problem-solving approach.

Firm Insistence and Acceptance of Anger

It is important to convey to depressed people that you think they can do the task. Often, by firmly insisting that they do so, you will evoke their anger. If you remember that depression can be viewed as anger turned inward, you will not be put off by its expression. In fact, you will realize that anger is healthier than withdrawal, and is a sign of progress in the depressed person.

The Nurse's Need to Be Liked

Unfortunately, what is potentially helpful to the client often gets merged with our own needs to be liked. It is possible to be helpful to clients without having them like us or our actions. In order to be helpful to depressed clients, you first need to become aware of what reactions they evoke in you. Common responses are anger, chronic helpfulness, and helplessness. It is not unusual for a nurse to throw up his or her hands in exasperation, to always do things *for* a depressed person, or to end a visit nearly in tears and with the words, "I give up. This person does not want my help." These responses are real and are to be expected when one is confronted by a depressed person who may go over and over faults, who seems to take forever to accomplish a task, or who may never implement your advice. What is useful about being able to identify your reactions to a transaction with a depressed person is that many of your feelings probably mirror his; he feels angry and impotent too.

Once you have identified your feelings, you can move on to the next task, which is examining your need to be liked. Sometimes your own needs get in the way of your helping clients meet their needs. Table 4-3 lists some realistic

Table 4-3 Examining Your Work Goals

Unrealistic work goals	Realistic work goals
To be needed by all clients	To identify clients or clients' problems that you have difficulty or success working with
To be liked by all clients	To test out nursing interventions and find ones that work
To master impossible situations	To feel satisfied that you've structured your day and applied all your skills and knowledge to solving the problems of clients
To be approved of by all clients	To learn about clients and about new procedures for helping clients
To have clients feel sorry for you	To be able to accept the angry responses of your clients as useful for them
To have clients meet your needs	To find ways outside of the nurse-client relationship and professional situation of meeting your own needs for learning and approval

and unrealistic work goals. If your goals are unrealistic, it is important to find new ones that are less likely to result in your feeling frustrated and helpless.

SUICIDE AND HOMICIDE

People who contemplate *suicide* do so because they see no alternative ways of making their lives more satisfying. They frequently have lost communication with their families and friends, and may use a suicide attempt as a symbolic way of saying, "I need help."

Suicide, like most violent actions, elicits a host of strong feelings in helpers, including anger, guilt, and helplessness. There may be excessive feelings of guilt and helplessness ("How could I let this happen?") alternating with feelings of anger ("What a stupid thing to do, trying to kill yourself!") It is interesting that helpers' feelings seem to follow the pattern of the grief process, and yet it is not surprising since death (or potential death) is a loss, and is thus expected to elicit a grief reaction.

There are certain groups of people that appear to have a higher suicide potential than others do (Schneidman and Mandelkorn, 1967; Seiden, 1974; Smith, 1976). These are people who:

1 Have a specific suicide plan
2 Are unemployed
3 Are unable to see alternatives
4 Lack communication with significant others

5 Have a history of suicide attempts
6 May be just coming out of a depression
7 Are overwhelmed by stress
8 Have a chronic, debilitating condition
9 Are over age 50 (if white)
10 Are age 15 to 44 (if black)
11 Are male rather than female
12 Have no religious ties
13 Want to be reunited with a dead significant other person
14 Report constant pain
15 Hear voices telling them to kill themselves
16 Take hallucinatory drugs (that encourage risk taking)
17 Use alcohol, barbiturates, or both

In addition to assessing the presence of these high-potential suicide predictors (the more predictors that are present, the higher the potential) you should be aware that it is a myth that people who talk about suicide never commit it. Chances are that by accident, if not on purpose, people who have characteristics predictive of suicide will succeed in killing themselves or in provoking others to kill them. In some cases, there may be no way to prevent them from doing so.

If you have any idea or feeling that clients may be thinking of killing themselves or others, you should encourage them to discuss these matters openly with you. Since feeling cut off from others and being unable to communicate can lead a person to consider suicide, your merely talking with such a person may offer a partial solution to his problem. It is also wise to tell him that you cannot keep this information to yourself since you cannot be responsible for his total care or for his life. It is important for you to share with others your knowledge of a person's suicidal or homicidal thoughts and feelings for a number of reasons. First, it is your responsibility as a nurse to promote healthy behaviors. Second, the guilt that can result from bearing the responsibility for such knowledge by yourself can be overwhelming; if the suicide or homicide should actually occur, guilt may be paralyzing. Third, when people contemplate suicide, they need as many realistic supports as possible; you are one source of support, yet you cannot always be there. Therefore, family and friends need to be encouraged to share the responsibility for those who feel helpless. Some suicidal messages are indirect, e.g., making offhand statements such as, "Life isn't worth living" or suddenly writing a will.

Suicidal feelings are easier to deal with than homicidal feelings since the latter may lead to a criminal offense and may have legal ramifications for you. Therefore, once a person confides in you that he or she may kill another person, you could legally be regarded as an accessory. Therapists who work with homicidal people deal with this dilemma in the following way: the client is told not to reveal any information that may be incriminating because the therapist would then have to share any knowledge of such illegal activities with the authorities. You will very likely not have to work with a homicidal person, although you may work with many suicidal people. Once a client communicates (either directly or indirectly) that he or she is thinking of suicide, you can help to clarify this communication. Some comments that you may make are: "Are you thinking of killing yourself?" or "Have you been thinking about suicide?" If the person answers, "Yes," you should then pursue this line of questioning with, "What are your thoughts?" "Have you a plan?" "Have you ever made a suicide attempt?" If the client has made a previous suicide attempt, get the particulars; stabbing oneself in the chest or trying to shoot oneself are more potentially lethal methods of suicide than taking two aspirin. The more potentially lethal the attempt, the higher is the potential for suicide.

Next, it is important to tell the client, "This is important material that needs to be shared with your family or friends; how would you like to broach the subject with them?" and "How can I help?"

Once you have clarified your own feelings and responsibilities, it will be easier for you to approach this topic in a neutral way and view it as another nurse-client problem to solve. If you feel confused or highly anxious, it is best to seek immediate mental health nursing consultation and/or assistance from a crisis intervention team. In general, the following nursing interventions can be used when working with people who threaten or attempt suicide.

1 Examine your own anxiety and guilt. Place the suicidal behavior in perspective. You may not have been given sufficient information by the client or family to assess suicidal potential accurately.

2 Bring the behavior out into the open and discuss it with the suicidal person and as many family members or friends as possible. For example, you might say something like, "Your wife told me you tried to stab yourself with a knife. What is this all about?" or "It's important to realize that Tom tried to kill himself and may be feeling isolated and cut off from you right now."

3 Place responsibility for the suicidal person's behavior on his or her family and friends. Suggest that they call a family meeting to deal with this problem. Some useful comments at this point might be: "When people try to take their life it is often a plea for help. It is important to rally around now and plan how your family (friends) can support and communicate more openly with Susan."

4 Suggest options to family members, e.g., specific times for the suicidal person to talk with them openly about his or her feelings. These times should be written down so that the suicidal person will have a concrete, future event to look forward to. Suggest ways to involve clergy, friends, and others in a support system for the suicidal person at this time. Call or tell the family to call the suicide hotline or crisis intervention team from the local community mental health center. Tell the family that a suicidal crisis usually lasts only 48 to 72 hours, and that open communication and support are crucial during that time. Counsel family members to take the suicidal person's threat seriously. Tell them that it is not true that people who talk about killing themselves seldom do it.

Help the family to evaluate its level of stress and ability to deal with a family member who constantly threatens or attempts suicide. For example, help family members to discuss the pros and cons of brief hospitalization, nursing home residency, and long term counseling and/or psychotherapy for the family.

CHILD ABUSE

Child abuse is a learned pattern of behavior. Parents who abuse their children were usually abused by their parents. Abused children are not necessarily unwanted children, but they are often those who cause their parent(s) to feel trapped and pressured by such behaviors as crying, whining, and constantly demanding. In large families, the parent in question may single out one child as the scapegoat and abuse him or her (Shanus, 1975). Children or infants may evoke an abusive response because they seem unsatisfied no matter what the parent does.

It is common to find ineffective relationships existing between parents in families where child abuse occurs. Unwed, adolescent mothers and even married, adult mothers whose relationship with their spouse is not satisfying may turn to the child as their sole source of love. Thus, the cry or unaffectionate behavior of the child may be interpreted as rejection and hostility by them. Other parents may act as if they expect the child to take care of them, and the child's refusal to do so may trigger their rage and hostility. Hopkins (1970) found that abusive parents are suspicious of and isolated from others with no source of support from neighbors or friends.

The definition of child abuse varies. Severely battered children are quite easy to identify. Children who are not sufficiently fed or clothed are also being abused. Finally, children who are constantly being told that they are unwanted and unloved or unlovable are also suffering from abuse because their self-image and self-esteem have been damaged.

Morris (1966, p. 11) has identified the following characteristics of rejecting behavior that mothers show toward their infants that can be noticed within the first few weeks of the mother-child relationship and that indicate high potential for abuse and neglect:

- Seeing the infant as ugly
- Perceiving the infant's odor, vomitus, feces, urine, drooling, or sucking as revolting
- Preoccupation or annoyance with odor, consistency, and number of infant stools
- Holding the infant roughly or without adequate support, or picking up the infant suddenly, without verbal or physical warning
- Worrying about infant's natural motor activity or relaxation
- Avoiding eye contact with the infant and/or staring fixedly at him or her
- Not talking to or cooing at the infant

- Making comments about the infant being unloving, being defective, being judgmental, or having a fatal disease
- Demanding constant reassurance that the infant is normal
- Not being able to discriminate between the infant's signals of hunger, fatigue, and need for stimulation or contact
- Either inadequately or excessively meeting the infant's immediate needs

Freidman (1976) has listed several factors that can alert you to the possibility that child abuse is occurring. The abused child has an unexplained injury or seems underfed, is unusually fearful, tries to take care of parents' needs, is different in physical or emotional makeup from other family members, and is dressed inappropriately. Shanus (1975) notes that in school abused children may be those who are disruptive, shy, complaining, who hang around after school, or who are always tired.

Freidman (1976) has listed the following characteristics that are common to abusive parents: feelings of loss of control, presenting contradictory history, projecting blame on others, having a seemingly detached manner, misusing drugs or alcohol, having a history of being abused as a child, showing reluctance to give information, having unrealistic expectations of the child, having no one to go to when feeling pressured by the child's demands, refusing consent for diagnostic studies for the child, and ignoring and/or being extremely inpatient with the child's demands.

Assessing and Intervening in Child Abuse

In assessing the potential for child abuse, it will be somewhat helpful for you to know certain high risk factors. Young mothers who have children close in age or who have no source of interpersonal support, parents married or single who have a history of substance abuse or delinquency, who have been raised in an abusive environment, who produce a handicapped or premature child (National Conference on Child Abuse, 1973), who are poor, who are having their first child, or who have a firstborn of the opposite sex have a greater potential for child abuse (Morris, 1966).

Paulson (1976) has focused his work on child abuse as a symptom of family breakdown. He has isolated a cluster of factors that seem to be predictive of child abuse: violence in parents' own childhood; ineffective communication patterns between parents; impulsiveness in parents; withdrawn, hyperactive, or colicky behavior in the child; and a particular stress event or factor such as a minor misbehavior by the child that triggers the abuse.

Steinmitz and Strauss (1973, p. 53) report that "If the social system does not provide an individual with the resources needed to maintain his or her family position, that individual will use violence if he is capable of it." They found evidence to support the idea that husbands who were inadequate providers or who felt dissatisfied with their jobs were much more likely to use violence, including corporal punishment of their children. In these homes, repressed intra-family conflicts erupt into violence. A preventive intervention in such homes would be to teach family members how to disagree without attacking each other, how to accept each other's differences, and how to talk about rather than act out their feelings. Such teaching would require the expertise of a clinical specialist in psychiatric-mental health nursing or of a professional person with a similar background. When you came across such families, you can refer them to the appropriate helper or agency.

It is useful to be aware of parents' knowledge of, expectations of, and inter-actions with their offspring. Recognizing disguised appeals for help is part of your job. Mothers who appeal for help in diapering infants, who indicate a lack of parenting skills, or who show those signs of rejection listed by Morris (1966) are indicating that they lack knowledge, and need help. You may have to teach parents how to make eye contact with and how to give appropriate amounts of sensory stimulation to their infants. These behaviors may, at first glance, seem obvious. Although they may seem so to you, they are not obvi-ous to parents or they would have already been implemented. Parents may need to be instructed in how to teach their children, how to set effective limits, and how to view crying as communication; they may need to be taught that children are not adults who can be expected to take care of their parents, and that children cannot be spoiled by getting loving attention. Gordon's *Parent Effectiveness Training* (1975) is one of several sources that you could use to teach clients in this area.

Interviewing and the use of questionnaires are other ways to collect informa-tion on child-parent relationships. Some questions Hopkins (1970) suggests are: "When your child cries, what do you do?" "If that doesn't work, what do you do?" "What happens if you are unable to stop your child from crying?" "Does your child sleep well?" "What do you do when he doesn't sleep?" and "Whom have you turned to for help?" Questionnaires are currently being used in pre- and postnatal clinics, obstretric units, well baby clinics, and outpatient depart-ments to detect parental needs and to identify high risk parents before abuse or neglect occurs. Families in which there is a premature, low birth weight infant, or an infant with a physical defect, should automatically be tagged for pre-ventive counseling on parenting skills, their feelings about the child, and the tendency to scapegoat a child who is different (Freidrich and Boriskin, 1976).

Prenatal clinic waiting time can be used to expose parents to child develop-ment material via audiovisual aids and group discussion. Prenatal education should include reality orientation to both the joys and problems of having and rearing a child. Such instruction can serve to lessen any unrealistic expectations that parents may have of the child as a potential parent or source of support for them.

Zalba (1971) suggests that preventive mental health services should be offered to the family at its most obvious points of stress, such as:

- When the first child is born
- When a parent loses a job
- When the first child enters school
- When the second child is born
- When the first child of the opposite sex is born
- When a family member enters or leaves the home
- When a family member contracts a chronic illness

Because many people, including nurses, think that offering such a service implies that the client is crazy or sick there is great resistance to this idea. Both you and your potential clients can gain much by your presenting this kind of service in a positive light since it can be helpful in preventing later difficulties. One way to present this kind of service to potential clients is to say, "I'm talking with you because we have discovered that the birth of a first child (or whatever stressor is under consideration) can be a particularly stressful event in the life of the family. So, I want to offer you assistance at this time of adjustment for you. What has been your experience (thoughts, feelings, expectations) so far?"

Nurses who work in hospital settings are beginning to take a stand against routine discharge of infants in the care of mothers who have nowhere to go, who have no one to be with them in the home, or who exhibit any of the patterns of rejection identified by Morris (1966). Like people who are about to commit violent acts such as suicide or homicide, potentially abusive parents frequently ask for help in indirect and even in direct ways. When these requests for help are rebuffed by "promises, preachments or evasions" (Morris, 1966), parents may have no other alternative but to release their anger and frustration on one of the nearest objects to them, their child. For these reasons, active listening and rapid intervention on your part can be crucial.

You can also take steps to reassure mothers about their infants. As part of this process, you must decipher the meaning behind their questions. If a mother refuses to accept that her infant is healthy, you need to explore further her potential for abusive behavior by gathering the information suggested above.

Nursing visits need to be continued in the home after high-risk mothers have been discharged from the hospital with their infants. Relief caregivers may be needed to help the parents and to take the pressure off of them. The use of relatives alone as relief caregivers is not recommended because it can create additional stresses among family members (Freidman, 1976). Supportive services from professional as well as from nonprofessional sources should be included in such a health care program. Parents Anonymous, a self-help group for abusive parents, is one nonprofessional support structure available. Crisis nurseries have been established in some parts of the country; these nurseries provide a safe place where parents can temporarily leave their children when they feel they may abuse them. Twenty-four hour telephone crisis lines and parent aid groups are additional sources of support for abusive parents that can be established if they do not already exist in the community.

Shanus (1975) reports the work of Dr. Henry Kempe at the National Center for Prevention of Child Abuse and Neglect in Denver, Colorado. Dr. Kempe estimates that 90 percent of abusive parents may be treated by reconstituting their sense of trust and by giving them moment-to-moment support over a 8- to 9-month period. He has found it unnecessary to remove the abused child from the home and to place him or her in a foster or adoptive home. Only 10 percent of abusive parents use the child as a scapegoat; in these cases, removal of the child from the home is suggested. Since it may be difficult for you to recognize which group parents fall into, it is wise to refer abusive parents to local community mental health centers, family counseling clinics, or to a clinical specialist in psychiatric-mental health nursing.

Other health services are also being developed. For example, temporary living quarters where mothers (usually single women) can stay with their children and where can they learn the basics of child care, cooking, and shopping, as well as develop trust and complete their education, have been established in some communities. These temporary living situations offer shelter to "hard-core parents who in most cases have killed a child" (Fontana, 1976, p. 6).

After you have assessed and intervened in child abuse, it may be helpful to evaluate your effectiveness. Some of the guidelines to follow in this self-evaluation (Helfer, 1973) are:

- Have parents developed an ability to use others in time of need?
- Have parents developed interests outside of the home?
- Is one parent able to recognize when the other needs help and see to it that he or she receives such help?
- Have parents resolved basic crises such as those in the areas of housing, nutrition, employment, illness, or relationships with in-laws?
- Are obstacles to achieving help minimal (e.g., is the phone operating and is transportation available)?
- Do parents view the child as different or as a potential parent or appendage to them?

YOUR FEELINGS

Perhaps the most important facet of your intervention in grief, depression, suicide, homicide, or child abuse is your own feelings about these behaviors. If you have feelings of anger, disgust, and/or avoidance, or see parents as victimizers and children as victims, you will not be effective. Therefore, it is essential that you are able to view the entire family system. For example, in cases of child abuse you need to be able to identify how deprivations that the parents suffered at the hands of their own parents or siblings or how the perceived differentness or crankiness of an infant may have provoked abusive responses in the parents. This sorting-out process may be initiated on an individual basis. Eventually, you will probably want to meet with other community health nurses to share your feelings and approaches. Also, you may occasionally want to include a psychiatric mental health nursing specialist as a consultant or facilitator for these discussions. Since your feelings around grief, depression, and violent behavior may be strong, it would help you to gain perspective as well as support for your practice by including a more objective nurse in your meetings.

SUMMARY

Grief is the expected response to a loss. Depression can be viewed as the result of frustration and hostility being turned inward. Depression can result when there is failure to grieve or as a result of learned helplessness. Suicide, homicide, and child abuse are external ways of coping with frustration and anger. It is possible to identify groups of people that have a higher potential for violent behavior than others do and to provide appropriate interventions.

PRACTICE EXERCISES

1 Examine Table 4-1 and add your own contributions to each of the three categories.
2 Assess your own grief responses by asking yourself the questions listed in Figure 4-1.
3 Devise a structured task chart for a depressed client; use Table 4-2 as your guide.
4 Using Table 4-3, examine your work goals; identify and reject your unrealistic work goals.
5 Identify your own feelings toward people who are depressed, suicidal, homicidal, or who abuse their children. Think of ways to handle your feelings so that you can be an effective helper.

REVIEW

Multiple-Choice Questions

1 Choose the individual below who has the highest potential for suicide.
   a A 60-year-old black female who has no specific suicide plan.
   b A 30-year-old white male who mixes alcohol and barbiturates and who is Catholic.
   c A 74-year-old woman whose husband has just died, who reports that she is in constant pain, and who wants to be reunited with her husband.
   d A devout Quaker who is unemployed and who has just been diagnosed as having multiple sclerosis.

2 Choose the situation(s) below that has (have) a high potential for child abuse.
  a A parent views the infant as ugly, revolting, defective, or annoying.
  b A child is disruptive or plays the role of peacemaker.
  c An infant is whiney, cries a lot, or has colic.
  d Parents have been abused themselves, misuse alcohol or drugs, have unrealistic expectations of the child, or have no source of interpersonal support.

Listing

1 List four interventions for learned helplessness.

_____

_____

2 List four interventions for a person who expresses suicidal thoughts.

_____

_____

_____

Matching Terms

Match nursing interventions with the stages in the grief process by placing the correct letter in front of the appropriate intervention.

Nursing intervention

1 _____ teach a new procedure

2 _____ remain present and decrease the patient's sensory input

3 _____ be available, and reflect or encourage the patient's anger

4 _____ sit silently with the client and note his or her nonverbal signals of isolation and loneliness

Grief process stage

a shock, disbelief

b anger

c denial

d acceptance

REFERENCES

Beck, A. et al. 1975. Hopelessness and suicide behavior: an overview. *Journal of the American Medical Association* 234, 11(December 15):1146–1149.

Bishop, B. 1976. A guide to assessing parenting capabilities. *American Journal of Nursing* 76, 11:1784–1787.

Carlos, N. 1975. Coping with newly diagnosed blindness. *American Journal of Nursing* 75, 12:2161–2163.

Carter, B. et al. 1975. Mental health nursing intervention with child abusing and neglecting mothers. *Journal of Psychiatric Nursing* 13:11–15.

Cherry, R., and Cherry, L. 1973. Depression. *New York Times Magazine* November 25, pp. 115–135.

Colgrove, M. et al. 1976. *How to survive the loss of love: 58 things to do when there is nothing to be done.* New York: Lion Press.

Coyne, J. 1976. Depression and the response of others. *Journal of Abnormal Psychology* 85, 2:186–193.

Eastwood, M. et al. 1975. Suicide, diagnosis and age. *Canadian Psychiatric Association Journal* 20, 6:447–449.

Fontana, V. 1976. New York hospital develops model program in child abuse. *Behavior Today* 7, 20:6.

Freidman, A. et al. 1976. Nursing responsibility in child abuse. *Nursing Forum* 15, 1:95–112.

Freidrich, W., and Boriskin, J. 1976. The victim's role in child abuse. *Behavior Today* 7, 44:2–3.

Gordon, T. 1975. *Parent effectiveness training.* New York: Plume.

Helfer, R. 1973. *Making the diagnosis of child abuse and neglect.* Pediatric Basics, no. 10, Fremont, Mich.: Gerber.

Hooker, C. 1976. Learned helplessness. *Social Work* 21, 3:568–571.

Hopkins, J. 1970. The nurse and the abused child. *Nursing Clinics of North America* 5, 4:589–598.

Miller, J. 1976. *Toward a new psychology of woman.* Boston: Beacon.

Minuchin, S. et al. 1975. A conceptual model of psychosomatic illness. *Archives of General Psychiatry* 32, (August):1031–1038.

Morris, M. 1966. Psychological miscarriage: an end to mother love. *Trans-Action* 3, 2:8–13.

National Conference on Child Abuse. 1973. Rockville, Maryland: National Institute of Mental Health.

Paulson, M. 1976. New facility for battered children to emphasize family unit. *Behavior Today* 7, 38:4.

Rosen, D. 1976. The serious suicide attempt. *Journal of American Medical Association* 235, 19:2105–2109.

Seiden, R. H. 1974. Suicide: preventable death. *Public Affairs Report* 15, 4:1–5.

Seligman, M. 1975. *Helplessness: on depression, development, and death.* San Francisco: Freeman.

Shanus, B. 1975. Child abuse: a killer teacher can help control. *Phi Delta Kappa* 57, 7:479–482.

Shneidman, E. S., and Mandelkorn, P. 1967. *How to prevent suicide.* Public Affairs Pamphlet # 406. New York: Public Affairs Committee.

Smith, D. 1976. Adolescent suicide: a problem for teachers? *Phi Delta Kappa* 57, 8:539–542.

Spinetta, J. et al. 1975. Death anxiety in the outpatient leukemic child. *Pediatrics* 56, 6:1035–1037.

Steinmitz, S., and Strauss, M. 1973. The family as cradle of violence. *Society* 10, 6:50–56.

Swigar, M. et al. 1976. Grieving and unplanned pregnancy. *Psychiatry* 39, 1:72–80.

Zalba, S. 1971. Battered children. *Trans-Action* 8, 9–10:58–60.

Znanieckilopata, H. 1975. On widowhood: grief work and identity construction. *Journal of Geriatric Psychiatry* 8, 1:41–55.

Chapter 5

Family System Assessments

LEARNING OBJECTIVES

When you finish this chapter, you should be able to:

- Identify systems concepts
- List qualities that are characteristic of effective families

Community health nurses are more likely to work with the family as a whole than are nurses who work in hospitals. Because much of your work will be with families, you may do this work in the home of your clients. Working with families, and especially working with families on their own turf, has advantages as well as disadvantages (Speck, 1964).

One of the major advantages of working with families is that it gives you the opportunity to observe how family members learn and perpetuate healthy and unhealthy behaviors. It will be much less easy for you to see one family member as victim or victimizer or as patient or caretaker. By looking at the family as a unit, you will be able to see healthy and unhealthy aspects, and strengths and weaknesses in all family members. Family theorists seldom view one family member as the patient. It will also be helpful for you not to label the person who has been referred for treatment as the patient. This person may have been identified as the patient, but may actually be much healthier in certain ways than some other family members. For this reason, it is helpful to call the person who has been referred for treatment the *identified patient*, or *IP*, but not to assume that the focus of nursing assessment and intervention will be on that person.

You are even better able to view the interplay of family members when you work with clients in their home. Being in the home enables you to get some idea of the physical and emotional climate surrounding the family. When you see family members in a hospital or clinic, their behavior will be somewhat different than when they are at home because they are in a different interactional context, and especially because in this instance they are the visitors. Working with a family in the home also makes you privy to information that might be omitted or censored were you to see that same family in a clinic. Some of this valuable information includes: how parents deal with their children on a day-to-day level; how the external, physical aspects of the home environment add or detract from the family's healthy functioning; how pets influence the interaction of family members; how the family prepares and eats its food; how the family handles matters related to excretion and sexuality; and how the family prepares for holidays such as Christmas, and for events such as camp and vacations.

Another advantage of visiting families in their home is that you will see many clients who are not willing to go to an office, clinic, or hospital for help. Their reluctance to do so is understandable since hospitals and clinics are often associated with illness, whereas living in the community with one's family implies that one is well and functioning. Because of the tendency to think in these terms, clients who come to clinics or hospitals are less likely to form a therapeutic alliance with you, and may be highly suspicious and distant when you talk with them. When a family is seen in its own environment, i.e., the home, therapeutic alliances are often easier to establish. In addition, there may be clients who are physically or emotionally homebound and, in these cases, home treatment may be the most practical.

A major disadvantage of working with a family is that the interrelationships are more complex than the one-to-one relationship is. At times, so much will seem to be happening that, as a result, you may experience high anxiety when dealing with families. Also, it will be easy for you to play roles in the client family similar to those you play in your own family. Such an evocation of your own familial role by the family you are working with is an example of *countertransference*. Everyone has sensitive areas and/or blind spots in their relationships with others. It is important to examine and be aware of your own patterns of countertransference. One way to do this is to ask yourself the following questions.

- Do I seem especially attracted to or repulsed by one family member?
- Do I tend to play peacemaker when working with families?
- Do I become an ally to certain family members and not to others?

- Do I take messages back and forth between one family member and another?
- Do I jump in and give my opinion before encouraging family members to give theirs?
- Do I tend to do *for* family members rather than encourage them to do *for* themselves?

Another disadvantage of working with families, and especially of working with families in their own homes, is that there may be disruptions and in order to handle them you will have to be very flexible. It is difficult to control what happens when a family is interviewed at home; dogs may growl, children may interrupt, spouses may argue, the family may tell you to leave or may not even let you in. When seeing families in their home, it is important for you to consider the issue of territoriality. In your office or clinic, you set the tone and establish the structure of the interview, move chairs to accommodate your clients, and so on. When you are in the clients' territory, they assume control of objects and relationships. It is their turf and, as such, you need to be careful not to move important family objects or possessions, to sit in the armchair usually reserved for the head of the house, or to refuse social offerings such as coffee or a cold drink. There may be times when you will assume control in all these areas, but it is important to first assess when such interventions are helpful to the family, and not to confuse this control with interventions that serve to relieve your own anxiety.

SYSTEMS THEORY

A *system* can be defined as a complex of components in mutual interaction (Von Bertalanffy, 1966). A *systems approach* focuses on interactional processes rather than on individual behavior, and on circular causality rather than on linear causality. In *circular causality*, no one person is to blame for a behavior occurring and recurring; rather, the behavior is seen as being reinforced and evoked by oneself and by others.

A family is an example of an *open system*. Open systems exchange information or matter/energy with their environments (Miller, 1969). For example, you can talk to families and exchange information with them. Open systems are only partially open to this exchange; they tend to move toward a stable, steady state where the status quo is maintained. If you try to introduce too much information or change into a family system, disorganization may occur and its steady state will be disrupted. At times, this disorganization may be the preferred intervention. Family therapists often spend years trying to influence families to change. Although you may fear changing a family, it is very difficult to do so since families are highly resistant to change. Families tend to develop rigid and repetitive patterns of interaction. Dysfunction and disruption of its steady state can occur, however, when the family cannot adapt to a critical event such as the birth of a child, the death of a parent, an acute illness, or some other biological, social, economic, or political change.

The family has its own feedback system where part of what happens in the family (output) is contingent on the repetition and reintroduction of information about family functioning (Jackson, 1971). For example, the family may follow a pattern where the mother and father argue, are interrupted by the child, proceed to yell at the child, and then shift their focus to the child and his or her misbehavior. The pattern may then repeat itself and follow each argument. This example demonstrates how the behavior of each family member affects and is affected by the behavior of every other person in the family.

The way you communicate with a family (input) can have the effect of increasing the family's disorganization, decreasing its disorganization, or reinforcing its steady state. *Positive feedback* leads to a change or adaptation in a system (Watzlawick, 1967). Teaching patients, seeing family members individually as a way to help them become less identified and involved with each other, and directing families to behave in new ways are examples of positive feedback. *Negative feedback* leads to a steady state and the maintenance of stable relationships. Providing support to family members and encouraging them to share their thoughts and feelings with one another are examples of negative feedback.

For you to understand how a particular family functions, you must study the nature of that family system including its input and feedback mechanisms. Each family develops its own system of operating. Some families can cope with severe crises and can actually benefit from them while other families seem unable to cope with seemingly insignificant problems.

Perhaps the easiest family system to study is the marital system. Marriage is a complex unit composed of the male system, the female system, and the marital system, which results from the interaction of the male and female systems. It is a good example of the whole being more than the sum of its parts (Lederer and Jackson, 1968). There are a number of basic marital systems that can develop. One is a system in which husband and wife have areas in common where they work together, and areas where each functions independently of the other. Another system is one in which the husband or wife has independent activities while the other spouse centers all of his or her activities on the other; in this system, there is great potential for one spouse to feel left out of the other's activities. Another system is one in which both spouses are involved only in activities with one another; in this system, there is great potential for over-involvement with each other and for insufficient extramarital support systems to develop. There are, of course, variations on these themes, but you may want to use these three marital systems as reference points when you begin making family assessments.

While examining marital systems, you may also look for types of male-female relationships. Basically, there are two kinds: complementary and symmetrical (Lederer and Jackson, 1968). In a *complementary* relationship, two people exchange different types of behavior. The behaviors complement each other or they fit together, e.g., one gives and the other receives, or one teaches and the other learns. In a complementary relationship, one person is in the primary or authority position while the other is in the secondary or inferior position. During normal growth and development, the relationship with one's parents shifts from one that is complementary to one that is symmetrical. A *symmetrical* relationship is one in which two people exchange the same type of behavior. Each person initiates action, criticizes the other, offers advice, and shows tenderness. This type of relationship is apt to lead to competition unless both participants are comfortable with both giving and receiving. At times, one family member may indicate that he wants to change the nature of his relationship with another family member or with the family in general. If other family members are not ready for the shift in control and definition of family relationships that such a change would cause, they will prevail upon the initiator to lessen or modify that change. A common example of such an attempted change in family relationships is when a child reaches adolescence and attempts to be treated as an adult (symmetrical) and parents try to force the adolescent back into the child role (complementary).

The earlier relationships that each spouse had with members of his or her family will help to shape how they relate to each other. The child's position in the family as determined by age and his or her relationship with siblings of the opposite sex can have a major influence on how that child will relate to his or her eventual spouse. Toman (1976) has examined these relationships and has concluded that the most comfortable, least-conflicted marriage will be between an older brother of a sister and the younger sister of a brother (or vice versa). In such relationships, there are no conflicts over who is the senior partner or who is in charge of things, or over how one should relate to a peer of the opposite sex; each has the same peer relationship that he or she had in his or her primary family. Every possible sibling relationship can be examined in this way. The more the marital relationship differs from the preceding model, the more difficult each partner's adjustment will be. Toman has also examined the age gap between siblings and has found that siblings who are close in age have more conflict when they are young, but that they are also closer as adults. The one factor that seems to obscure the effect of these seniority/opposite sex experiences is the number of severe losses that is suffered by each child as he or she is growing up. Therefore, if you are privy to information about your clients' sibling relationships and losses of significant others, you will be able to anticipate some of their parenting and marital difficulties and you will also be able to understand why each parent relates to you in the way that he or she does. For example, if a younger brother of brothers marries a younger sister of sisters, both may look to the other for direction. Their children may also be looking for direction and leadership. Also, the husband may have some difficulty relating to you if you are a female, but no difficulty if you are a male, and especially if you are an older male.

Once a child is born, the marital system changes. Another person must be accommodated and relationships will change. In one family, husband and wife were having difficulty talking to each other without arguing and in showing tenderness to one another. When their first child was born, a shift in relationships occurred. Their communication pattern changed and conflict resulted. The wife-mother spent less time with her husband, thus decreasing the amount of conflict between them; instead she developed an intense relationship with her son. The husband had several options at this point, each of which had the potential for providing the system with positive or negative feedback and for influencing the behavior of the wife-mother and son, and vice versa. For example, the husband could have chosen to get upset, to spend more time at work, to drink with his friends, to find a substitute wife, to become more involved with his own parents, to wait until his wife was more available, to seek counseling assistance, to talk with his wife about his feelings, or to become more involved in the care of the child. Figure 5-1 shows some aspects of this family system and how it worked. In Figure 5-1, the husband gets involved outside of the

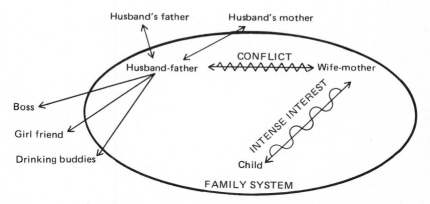

Conflict between the husband and wife is not dealt with directly. Instead, the husband looks for sources of support outside the marital system, while the wife becomes overinvolved with the child.

Legend:

<A^A^A> conflict

<A^A^A> intense interest; overinvolvement

<———> increased communication

Figure 5-1 How one family system works.

home, which leads to more anger and conflict between the spouses; the child now returns the intensity and warmth to the mother, thus gaining her attention and neutralizing parental conflict. If this pattern of using the child as a buffer or mediator between the parents were repeated a number of times, it might become a familiar way for the family to deal with parental conflict. As a result, the child may lose precious time from mastering his or her normal developmental tasks, but he or she will have helped to restore family homeostasis.

Another way that family systems maintain homeostasis or steady state is through the use of family myths. *Family myths* are beliefs that are shared by family members depiste the distortions of reality that such beliefs may engender. Myths are different from the social facade that the family as a group presents to you when you first meet it. The family myth is part of the way that the family appears to its own members; it is part of the inner image the family has of itself. In general, no one questions, challenges, or investigates whether the myth is true or real. The myth serves to explain the behavior of family members while it hides the motive for such behavior. Each family develops myths; you may or may not be privy to them. You may not be able to identify myths in some families because they are not revealed to you or because you have insufficient information to conclude that a myth is in operation.

In one family, whenever the husband did not pay attention to his wife, the wife-mother began to become overly concerned with her daughter's eating habits and to note how weak and sickly she was. By complaining to her husband about the daughter, the wife-mother was able to get his attention; meanwhile the daughter reinforced this pattern by eating only junk food and thus helped to maintain steady state. If the daughter had decided to eat a better diet or to move out of the house, the rest of the family might have focused on this behavior and have acted in ways to force the daughter to return to the more familiar pattern of family interaction (Ferreria, 1963). In this family, the myth that was perpetuated was that the daughter was sickly. The real family problem was that there was a lack of communication between husband and wife. Family myths serve to both obscure family problems and protect family members from difficulties that they feel unable to deal with directly.

The family system stabilizes itself through the use of a triangle which is "the smallest stable relationship system" (Bowen, 1971, p. 394). In periods of calm, two people in the three-person system are closer, while the third may be comfortable (or not so comfortable) as the outsider. The third person is constantly attempting to form a closer bond with one of the others (or with another person outside of the three-person system). There may be competition for attention, affection, warmth, or tenderness. In periods of stress, the outsider position is the most comfortable and desirable; now, each person moves to escape the two-person tension system. When it is not possible to shift forces in the triangle, a fourth person may be "triangled in," which leaves the third person free of the system at that moment. Families may try to triangle you in. Families have been known to relieve their tensions by projecting them on to outside workers. A family triangle in moderate tension has two comfortable relationships and one relationship that is in conflict. If you look at Figure 5-1, you can visualize a triangle by thinking of the line from husband-father to child as the side of the triangle; as tension increases, the husband-father may try to triangle in his own parents, boss, secretary, or others.

By refusing to side with one or the other parent, but by actively trying to listen to and understand each one, you can help to stabilize a family at a healthier level of functioning as each parent learns to differentiate and value him- or herself. All families use triangles. Healthy families triangle their members in and out in a fluid fashion; less healthy families have very rigid triangles that recur with predictable regularity.

Another way the family stabilizes itself is through prejudicial scapegoating (Ackerman, 1971). When conflict and/or anxiety rise to intolerable levels, warring factions within the family may focus their hostility on individual differences. Some individual differences that families may choose to attack are differences in physical appearance, personal attitudes, character traits, and moral values. Symbolic meanings are attached to these differences, and individual family members may view the person who is perceived as different as dangerous. This person then becomes the victim, and the family uses that person's behavior as a convenient source of blame whenever tension rises. The person who becomes the victim agrees on some emotional level to be vulnerable and attackable. Another person(s) in the family emerges as attacker, and a third as healer or peacemaker. Although this process may temporarily provide support and restore stability, in the long run, it leads to fragmentation and alienation (Ackerman, 1971). At times, families may attempt to get you to join in such prejudicial scapegoating and play the role of attacker or healer. You must guard against allowing yourself to be unwittingly drawn into family coalition. In order for this not to happen, you need to watch for signs of this dynamic operating in families with which you work.

Leininger (1973) has found a variant of the scapegoating phenomenon that explains why some families may use witchcraft practices to cope with problems related to acculturation. For example, she found that there was a displacement of intragroup stress onto the members of the outgroup, who were then referred to as witches. A victim was identified in the family or primary group and a medium or attacker was also located; the medium often turned out to be the mother or older sister of the victim. Leininger explains the witchcraft phenomenon as a way of resolving family problems related to value changes and ambivalence about changing traditional family relationships. As a community health nurse, you can begin to identify how families can participate in scapegoating one member and how cultural mechanisms can be used by families to regain family equilibrium.

SELF-ESTEEM AND FAMILY INTERACTION

Years ago, the family was the center of formal education, religious learning, and socialization. Today, the family provides the training ground for emotional learning and self-esteem. The responsibility for formal and religious education has been assumed by other institutions. At the same time as the functions of the family were decreasing, the size of the family was shrinking. Today, the extended family composed of grandparents, uncles, and aunts is uncommon. With a shrinkage in the size of the family has come an increased intensity of emotional reaction to other available family members. Since there are fewer people to relate with, fewer people must provide the necessary solace, instruction, support, and criticism. With this increase in intensity of relationships and decrease in available people to relate with has emerged a high degree of unrealistic expectation about what family members can hope to receive from and give to one another (Satir, 1975).

The family continues to be where most people learn self-esteem. It is within the family that people first learn to feel good or bad about themselves and their ability to live a satisfying life, as well as to learn how to differentiate themselves from other family members. In families that foster low self-esteem, family members are taught not to trust others, to be critical of their own and others' abilities, and to withdraw or attack others.

According to Satir (1964) mate selection in our society can be viewed from the vantage point of self-esteem. A person with low self-esteem has a greater sense of anxiety and uncertainty about himself. Therefore, he tends to be overly concerned about how others view him and is especially concerned about impressing others, disguising his needs, feeling inadequate and inferior, and maintaining strong ties to his own original family. Because of these factors, this person may have unrealistic expectations of his chosen mate but, at the same time, may trust his mate only minimally. Neither partner will be completely aware of these hopes and fears. If both partners have low self-esteem, their marital relationship will duplicate or be diametrically opposed to the relationship that each saw existing between their own parents. When these two people discover that they are different in ways that seem to detract from rather than add to their needs, the differentness that each sees in the other may be perceived as bad because it often leads to disagreement. Since many couples do not know how to resolve disagreement constructively, they tend to pretend that there are no differences and that both partners think, feel, and act the same on all issues. Certain areas of joint living constantly challenge all couples, but especially those who refuse to admit their differences. These are the areas of money, food, sex, recreation, work, child-rearing, and relationships with in-laws. When a couple is especially fearful of having differences, disagreements go underground (Satir, 1964) and become covert. Instead of saying, "I don't like it when you talk about me," indirect communication such as, "No one talks to me" may occur.

People who have low self-esteem may choose to have a child because they hope it will resolve their differences. Instead, the situation becomes more complex and the child may be asked to take on roles such as that of peacemaker, ally, messenger, or surrogate parent. In the peacemaker role, the child is expected to keep peace between the parents. In the ally role, the child is expected to side with one parent against the other. In the messenger role, the child is asked to take messages back and forth between parents who refuse to speak directly to one another. In the surrogate parent role, the child is asked by his mother or father to play his or her parent. All of these roles are beyond the capabilities of the child's level of growth and development and being forced to play one or all of them will leave the child insufficient time to complete his or her normal developmental tasks. It may also lead to resentment in the child, who may feel deprived of a normal childhood (Satir, 1964).

A child can also be encouraged in subtle ways to be a problem child. Parents who do this explicitly or outwardly criticize the child and at times punish him or her, yet at other times and in other ways they support the behavior in question. Such inconsistent behavior on the part of parents may take the form of failing to follow through on threats, delaying the child's punishment, acting indifferent to and accepting of the child's behavior, showing unusual interest in the behavior, or rewarding the behavior in indirect ways.

Children learn self-esteem when parents consistently demonstrate that they consider the child to be a person who can master the environment and show all aspects of self—sexuality, intelligence, tenderness, anger, and so on. In the functional family the mates are confident about their own survival and do not need to cling to one another or the child. Because neither parent worries about being left out, each can allow the child to develop a relationship with the other parent.

Children of parents who continually criticize them, who withdraw from them, who physically harm them, or who do not set and stick to firm guidlines for behavior are likely to have low self-esteem. Children tend to repeat the patterns of relating that they learned from their parents. These repeated, unhealthy patterns of behavior can be broken if family members are able to have satisfying relationships with significant other people outside of the family; at times, this significant other person could be you.

Each child in a family must somehow resolve the following issues effectively in order to differentiate him- or herself successfully from other family members (Satir, 1971).

- How can I feel masterful and powerful when my parents have so much power?
- How can I be independent in a situation where interdependence is required?
- How can I be a sexual person when this aspect of life is shrouded in secrecy?

- How can I be productive without being judged or valued primarily for producing?
- How can I share my thoughts and feelings without harming others?

When children who have not effectively resolved one or more of these issues grow up and marry, they transmit their own problems to their children by teaching them what they learned from their parents. In this way, low self-esteem is passed from generation to generation.

In the context of the larger system, families that have few or no effective relationships with other community members, that have a prevailing sense of helplessness, and that think others control their destinies are likely to be less effective (Satir, 1971).

ASSESSING FAMILY INTERACTION

There are characteristics of relationships and of relating to others that are for the most part considered to be functional. There are other characteristics that are not so functional. It will help you to learn how to differentiate relationships that are functional from those that are not so functional. In general, functional relationships are those in which members are confident about their ability to relate to one another; communication is clear and direct and feedback is asked for and responded to; disagreement can occur without belittlement; and others are treated as having the potential for being masterful, sexual people (Satir, 1964).

It is not always easy to tell if family members are relating effectively or if they have problems relating. In general, there are four areas of family functioning that you can study to determine this: productivity, leadership, communication, and conflict.

Effective families are able to achieve a balance between accomplishing a task and having fun while doing it. In problematic families there may be so much fooling around that little is accomplished, or there may be so much discipline and rigidity of behavior that work is very grim. For example, if the task is to plan a vacation, effective families will plan the vacation completely, and, at the same time, will be enthusiastic and have fun while planning.

Effective families have some form of leadership. It might be democratic or it might be dictatorial or it might be some other form. There is no one right type of leadership; each effective family system develops a form that suits it. In ineffective families, there is no clear form of leadership.

In effective families, the members speak clearly and openly to one another while in ineffective families the members find ways to avoid and interfere with clear communication. Effective families neither shy away from nor provoke conflict; the members realize that all families fight, but they do not go out and look for an argument. In ineffective families, the members either battle all the time, or pretend that they are in agreement all the time.

In general, effective families are able to accomplish necessary tasks without feeling grim and weary; the members can communicate their needs, wants, and wishes directly to one another and they can argue and disagree in a constructive fashion (Satir, 1975).

Van der Veen (1972) has found that some important questions to ask about family effectiveness are related to adaptive coping. *Adaptive coping* includes all of the ways in which the family adapts to the world around it. More effective families can build relationships with the community, can take risks or make ventures, and have a sense of control over their destiny.

Satir (1971) defines a *dysfunctional family system* as one in which the growth needs of individuals are not accommodated, the methods of achieving satisfactory joint outcomes are not available, and the ways of using the outside world to expand and change itself are not included. Bowen (1971) focuses mostly on families where members are not allowed to be individuals. In such cases, couples usually complain that they do not know why they stay together, but they do stay together for years. These families fight over everything but the real issues. Both spouses seem to be reasonable people until they are together, and then they are ruled by irrationality. He calls this type of family "the undifferentiated ego mass" (p. 395) because there is only a "we" family component, and no "I" or individual component is allowed to develop. It would seem that in effective families an individual sense of self as well as a sense of we-ness or being part of a unit is possible and even encouraged. Family system interventions are presented in Chapters 6 and 12.

SUMMARY

Treating the family on its own turf has both advantages and disadvantages. From the family systems perspective there is an identified patient, but all family members are considered to be part of any problem or effective level of functioning. Some assessments you can make are in the areas of complementary and symmetrical relationships, peer relationships in the parents' primary families, triangles, feedback, myths, scapegoating, levels of self-esteem, and of effective and ineffective family relationships.

PRACTICE EXERCISES

1 Make an evaluation of your own family in terms of triangles, feedback, communication patterns, leadership, and productivity.
2 Choose a family you do not know and attempt to get all the members together so that you can talk with them. You might choose to focus on a set of questions that you have prepared prior to visiting the family, or you might merely tell the members that you are there to learn about them and take it from there. Your task is to assess that family system by gathering as much information as you can about it.

REVIEW

Listing

List qualities that are characteristic of effective families.

_____

_____

_____

Matching Terms

Match system concepts with the examples by placing the correct letter in front of the appropriate system concept.

System concepts	**Examples**
1 _____ scapegoating	**a** the husband decides and the wife agrees
2 _____ family myth	**b** a particular child always gets blamed for things
3 _____ feedback	**c** the wife tries to get you to side with her
4 _____ triangling in	**d** the belief that arguing is harmful
5 _____ complementary relationship	**e** the giving and receiving of information

REFERENCES

Ackerman, N. 1971. Prejudicial scapegoating and neutralizing forces in the family group, with special reference to the role of "family healer." In *Theory and practice of family psychiatry*, ed. J. Howell, pp. 626-634. New York: Brunner/Mazel.

Barry, M. 1972. Feedback concepts in family therapy. *Perspectives in psychiatric care* 10:183-189.

Bowen, M. 1971. Family therapy and family group therapy. In *Comprehensive group psychotherapy*, eds. H. Kaplan and B. Sadock, pp. 384-420. Baltimore: Williams and Wilkins.

_____ 1972. Toward the differentiation of a self in one's own family. In *Family interaction: a dialogue between family researchers and family therapists*, ed. J. Framo, pp. 111-173. New York: Springer.

_____ 1976. Toward the differentiation of self in one's family of origin. Paper read at The Center for Family Learning, January 24, 1976, New Rochelle, New York.

Ferber, A. et al. 1973. *The book of family therapy*. Boston: Houghton Mifflin.

Ferreria, A. 1963. Family myth and homeostasis. *Archives of General Psychiatry* 9:457–463.

Goldberg, H. 1975. Home treatment. *Current Psychiatric Therapies* 15:253–258.

Jackson, D. 1971. The study of the family. In *Theory and practice of family psychiatry*, ed. J. Howell, pp. 111–130. New York: Brunner/Mazel.

Lederer, W., and Jackson, D. 1968. *The mirages of marriage*. New York: Norton.

Leininger, M. 1973. Witchcraft practices and psychocultural therapy with urban families. *Human Organization* 32:73–83.

Miller, J. 1969. Living systems: basic concepts. In *general systems theory and psychiatry*, eds. W. Gray, F. Duhl, and N. Rizzo, pp. 51-133. Boston: Little, Brown.

Satir, V. 1964. *Conjoint family therapy*. Palo Alto: Science and Behavior Books.

_____ 1971. Symptomatology: a family production. In *Theory and practice of family psychiatry*, ed. J. Howell, pp. 663–670. New York: Brunner/Mazel.

_____ et al. 1975. *Helping families change*. New York: Aronson.

Speck, R. 1964. Family therapy in the home. *Journal of Marriage and the Family* 26:72–76.

Toman, W. 1976. *Family constellation*. 3d ed. New York: Springer.

Van der Veen, F. et al. 1972. Higher order dimensions of the family concept. Paper read at the Institute for Juvenile Research, March 1972, Chicago.

Von Bertalanffy, L. 1966. General systems theory in psychiatry. In *The American handbook of psychiatry*. vol. 3. ed. S. Arieti, pp. 705–721. New York: Basic Books.

Chapter 6

Family System
Interventions

LEARNING OBJECTIVES

When you finish this chapter, you should be able to:

- List ways to define yourself in your own family of origin
- Identify appropriate strategies for conducting a family interview
- Identify techniques for encouraging family communication

Your first experience with families was with your own family. Because of the intensity and longevity of this relationship you have developed strong emotional ties to and biases against your family. All of us remain somewhat undifferentiated from our families. Most of us are not aware of how attached we are to our primary families. Because of these attachments few of us see our parents as people; we tend to either down- or upgrade them.

If you plan to do extensive work with families, it will help you to be more effective if you begin to define yourself in your own family. This will allow you to see yourself more clearly in relation to the families you hope to help. If you are not clear about what your role(s) and behavior is in your family of origin, you are apt to repeat that behavior with clients simply because it is familiar and tends to be automatic. A planned nursing intervention is one that is based on an assessment of the clients' needs. An automatic nurse response that is based on your needs may or may not meet the clients' needs. Defining yourself in your own family requires that you do research on the emotional systems in your family (Bowen, 1976). It is recommended by Bowen (1975) that you plan visits to your family since anyone who wishes to effectively help other families needs to have knowledge of his or her own family system. He recommends visits to one's own family for the purpose of establishing person-to-person relationships with each member. Although such interpersonal relationships may already exist, many family members spend much of their time talking about other people or things rather than talking with each other about their unique qualities as people. If you decide to do this as a long-term relationship study, you would be wise to find a coach or supervisor who has already had this type of experience with his or her own family.

The result of doing this kind of family work is that you will be better able to observe and control your emotional reactions to your own family as well as to families you will eventually work with. By being in better control of your own emotions, you will be less likely to side with particular family members or to cast certain family members in the role of victim or victimizer. Although you will probably never become completely objective, observing and interviewing your own family can help you to get beyond blame, anger, and guilt. In order for this excercise to work, you cannot tell the members of your family that you are studying them. By doing so, you would increase their resistance to relating with you on a person-to-person level and you would create even further distance between yourself and other family members. Your task is not to psychoanalyze, distance yourself from, or alienate your family; your task is to get to know each family member individually. To do this, you must see each person alone; e.g., you can take your father to lunch or take a walk with your mother. If you attempt to relate with a family member on a one-to-one basis with others present, triangles will develop, and you will be less able to focus on the person you are trying to get to know.

Bowen (1975) recommends that the next step in decreasing emotional reactiveness to your own family is to visit with members during periods of emotional upset such as illness, death, or holidays. When your family is not under stress, members will work hard to prevent emotional issues from surfacing; under stress, emotional issues will rise to the surface. At this step, the idea is for family members to learn not to form triangles, even though there may be strong family pressures to do so. Provoking a confrontation with any family member is also not recommended since there is liable to result a brief breakthrough followed by a backlash and increased distance being placed between you and the family. Once you are able to get some emotional distance from your own family, you will be much less likely to be triangled in by the families with which you work (Bowen, 1975).

As a student community health nurse you can begin to focus some of your energy on working with the well family. By doing this, you will encounter less resistance and interference from other professional people, and you will be able to institute preventive health measures because there will be less competition for the patient and less time will be taken up focusing on sickness and/or on chronic conditions. A good way to begin this work is to locate a family in the community that is willing to work with you for a period of several years. Many nurses work with families because the IP is referred to them. However, once one family member is labelled as *the* patient it is much more difficult to see how other family members might also benefit from your services. For this reason, students are often given the assignment of finding a family in the community that will agree to work with them. Such an approach has many advantages and a few disadvantages. The primary disadvantage is that you will feel uncomfortable and very anxious in an ambiguous, unstructured situation in which you will have little control, little status, and in which you will also risk rejection. Such potential disadvantages can be decreased by using prepractice methods such as simulations.

If you have been assigned the task of finding a family to work with you, you will need to think about effective ways of establishing a relationship with a family. One way is to present your work as a collaborative effort that will benefit both parties; you will learn and gain experience and, at the same time, will provide the family with helpful services. In one community health experience, students agreed to proceed in the following manner:

1 Knock on the door and say, "I'm _____ , a student nurse at _____ . I'm learning about and assisting with family health care. It's important that I find a family to work with that has children. Do you have any children?" (The discussion would be terminated at this point if there were no children in the family. The student would then decide whether or not to spend a few moments talking with the family member in exchange for having bothered him or her. If the discussion had been continued, step 2 would have been followed; if not, the student would have gone on to the next house.)

2 "I'd like to come and visit you _____ times over the next _____ years. During that time I'll be helping you with health care information and you'll be telling me a little bit about your family's health care needs."

Although the students anticipated complete rejection, few, if any, family members slammed the door in their faces. Instead, many family members were eager to be offered special attention, concern, and the potential for health care. Exactly how you work with a family is up to you and/or your instructor or supervisor. If you are a beginning family worker, your task may be basically one of observing, listening, and providing support and information. If you are a more experienced family worker, you may take a more active role as counselor or therapist.

Currently, the type of family that you will most commonly encounter is the one that has been referred to you by clients or family members themselves or by persons in authority such as teachers or employers who think that the family is in difficulty. In this case, your role might be somewhat different since the family (or at least part of it) has already agreed that it can use help and sees you as someone who may be helpful. Most family interviews that you conduct will be of this kind. However, the discussion that follows can also be useful when interviewing a family that you have engaged to work with you.

CONDUCTING A FAMILY INTERVIEW

There are differing viewpoints on what the focus of a family interview should be. It will naturally be different depending on whether you are trying to obtain a mental health history, attempting to help a family deal with a specific problem or symptom, or aiming to establish long-term family therapy or counseling. (The last two goals require additional training and supervision by an experienced family therapist before you attempt to pursue them with a family.)

If the object of the family interview is to gather information about the family system, you can use either a structured or an unstructured format. In the structured format, you ask each family member specific questions and may direct him or her to complete a specific task such as fill out a questionnaire or plan an activity. Some questions that you might ask if you are there for the purpose of learning about the family's attitude toward and behavior regarding health care are:

1 Who is in the family? Are all family members present? If not, where are the missing members? What are their ages? What pets are there in the family?

2 What does each family member do for recreation? What do family members do together for recreation? How was this decided?

3 Where do family members go for help when they feel ill? How did the family decide to go there? How does the family get there? What has been each member's experiences in getting health care when he or she has needed it?

4 What changes have there been in the family within the past 2 years?

A family interview will be most beneficial if as many family members as possible are there at the same time. This may require an evening visit, or a visit at a time that is mutually acceptable to both you and the family. Some family members may be resistant to the idea of their all sitting down together with you for an interview. To decrease this resistance, you can say something like, "I want to get everyone's ideas" or "It's important that I talk to the whole family about health care."

Although the suggested questions seem to focus on specific health behaviors, when they are explored or expanded upon they can also provide a wealth of information about how the family views itself, about how the family relieves tension and has pleasant experiences, about how much family members do alone and together, about how family decisions are made, about what community resources the family has and what contacts it has made, about the family's past experiences with health caregivers, and about certain critical events that may have influenced family functioning recently.

Another purpose for a family interview may be to ascertain the family's ability to cope with a normal developmental change or with an unexpected situation. While conducting the interview, you can also watch for verbal and nonverbal signs that indicate whether the family is becoming more or less positive about its opinion of you as a helping person. If the goal is to assess a family's reaction to the presence of a disabled child in its midst, the following questions may be asked:

1 Who in the family helps with _____'s care?

2 How have things changed in the family since _____ was born?

3 How do you think you've been managing?

4 What problems have you been having?

5 What problems do you anticipate?

6 Is _____ acting as you thought he or she would?

7 Tell me about _____'s childhood illnesses (hospitalizations, operations, clinic appointments, etc.)

8 How does _____ get along with father (mother, siblings, teacher, friends)?

9 How does _____ deal with upsetting situations? Can you give me an example?

10 How does _____ manage his or her activities of daily living?

11 How can I be helpful to you as a family?

If children are old enough to answer, some of the questions can be directed their way. You may also need to explain why you are interested in the answers, how you can be helpful, and what your expectations of working with the family are. While talking with the family about the specific questions, you can also be observing how the parents relate to the child (and vice versa), what levels of anxiety and grief are present, what areas of the child's behavior seem to be within the normal range, and you can also be considering what interventions may be needed. More specifically, you can observe whether the parents seem to over- or underprotect the child and whether family members seem to be in the shock, denial, anger, or acceptance stage of grieving for the child. Since parents of disabled children frequently have strong feelings about having produced an imperfect person, look for whether they seem to think it is their fault, due to genetics, poor judgment, or something inexplicable. Other parents may project the blame onto some external source, seeing the disabled child as God's punishment for their sins, or even as a result of poor medical or nursing care.

If you work better in an unstructured atmosphere, you may wish to meet with family members and then just react to whatever questions they might ask or to whatever behavior they might act out. For example, you might ask a mother who has brought her infant and older child to the well baby clinic to sit down and talk with you for a few minutes. During that time you can observe how the mother holds the infant and how she talks with or looks at it, as well as how the older child relates to the infant and mother and vice versa. You might begin the conversation by making such an open-ended inquiry as, "Tell me how you're managing" or you could ask the older child, "What do you think about having a brother (sister)?" The way you structure or do not structure a family interview will depend on its purpose and on your style of relating.

In addition to asking questions, you can get to know a family by constructing a family genogram (see Figure 6-1). A genogram is like a family tree, but it also contains information about family relationships and health concerns. The genogram can alert you to potential family health problems in a way that merely asking for a history of family illnesses will not. By looking at the family genogram in Figure 6-1, it is clear that the illnesses on Margaret's side of the family include multiple sclerosis (m.s.) and diabetes. Family illnesses on Oscar's side of the family include heart disease. In addition, this family has suffered many losses. It is not clear how many are unresolved. Questions you may ask yourself in order to prevent further upsets are:

"Has Oscar's death been properly grieved by the family?"
"What effect did the death of Amy and Harv have on the family?"
"Was Mona a substitute child for David and Margaret? If so, did all parties adapt successfully?"

Other information that can be gleaned from studying the genogram is that Margaret is a younger sister of a brother and has married an older brother of sisters, thus duplicating her sibling relationship in her primary family.

Based on the information gathered through the genogram plus your assessment of family strengths and weaknesses, you may refer this family to a nurse family therapist or counselor who can help its members to mourn its losses and thus decrease its potential for parenting difficulties. The family would, of course, have to agree to such a referral. However, once you have established rapport with the members of this family, it is more likely that they will accept your recommendation for referral if you can present it to them as a preventive measure, and not as an indication that they are sick or weak.

The genogram is a technique that can be used both as an assessment tool and as an intervention technique. For example, it can be used as an intervention technique when your goal is for the family to work on a project together. Giving the

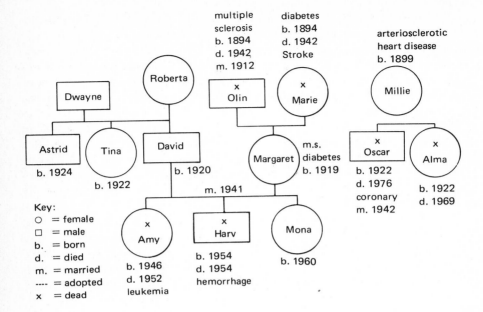

Key:
O = female
□ = male
b. = born
d. = died
m. = married
---- = adopted
x = dead

Guidelines for Constructing a Genogram

1 Obtain a large notebook or sketch pad with unlined paper.
2 Tell family members that one way that you gather information to help them is by drawing a special kind of family tree. If you decide that it will be helpful to the process, let them watch as you add information and/or ask them to add information to the genogram.
3 Begin by centering the names of the mother and father or IP in the middle of the page. Draw a circle around the name of a female and a square around that of a male. Insert the ages of the individuals in question in the appropriate circles or squares. Draw a line to connect a man (square) and a woman (circle) who are married. Write down the date of their marriage on the connecting line. Add lines perpendicular to the marriage line to indicate children. In this figure, Mona, Harv, and Amy are the children of David and Margaret.
4 Add extended family members such as parents of the spouses, important uncles, aunts, and so on.
5 Fill in important deaths, births, marriages, retirements, successes, physical illnesses, and so on.
6 Some questions that you can ask to gather this information are:
   "Let's see now, your first name is?" (Look at one spouse.)
   "And your name is?" (Look at the other spouse.)
   "You two were married in what year?"
   "You have three children. Their (your) names are?" "What are their (your) ages?"
   "What illnesses (diseases, operations, successful recoveries, permanent losses) have you each had?"
   "What did _____ die of?"
   "What was the effect on the family?"

Figure 6-1 Family genogram.

family a task such as filling in a genogram is not very threatening. In some instances, it can even bring family members closer together and may interest them in learning about their roots in a way that they have never been interested before.

If you are working with a family over a period of time, you can anticipate difficulties that may develop and plan special family visits or interviews around those times. The questions you ask or the activities you assign a family are chosen based on the purpose of the meeting or the anticipated difficulty. Hymovich (1974) suggests assessing the family's knowledge and plans whenever a new child is born or when a child is about to be hospitalized. Other critical times are when children or adolescents begin new school experiences or when other family members leave or enter the home. Sheehy (1976) has examined several predictable life crises of adulthood that may also serve as focal points for visits and family interventions.

ENCOURAGING FAMILY COMMUNICATION

In addition to the interview, there are certain techniques that you can use to encourage family members to communicate with you and with one another. Some of these are establishing rapport; using the family's language; encouraging democratic values; refraining from blaming or siding with family members; modeling clear, effective communication; eliciting alternate strategies for dealing with health problems; teaching family members how to disagree constructively and contract with one another.

Establishing Rapport

To establish rapport with a family, you must be aware of your own family's personal and cultural stereotypes. The family you visit will also have stereotypes of you as a nurse and as a member of a specific sociocultural background. These stereotypes will reveal themselves in the family's verbal and nonverbal communication; "How come a nurse is working with families? Where is the doctor?" or "How come you're interested in *my* family?" are examples of possible questions the family may ask you.

If you can present yourself in a nondefensive, clear way, it will be easier for you to establish rapport with a family. The two examples below illustrate how rapport was not established with the first family, but how rapport was established with the second family.

First Family
Nurse: I'm here to talk with you about your son, Romand. The school nurse suggested that I visit. Where shall we sit?
Mother: (looking puzzled) This is my brother, and these are my children.
Children: (in unison) Daddy, daddy. (as they run to the mother's brother)
Nurse: (puzzled) Your brother—or your husband?
Mother: Send someone else. You don't understand us. (as nurse is ushered out of the house)

Second Family

Nurse: I'm here to learn about your family and its health care.

Husband: What are you trying to do—put us under a microscope for study?

Nurse: Not really. I hope we can learn from one another.

Husband: What can we learn from you? You don't look old enough or smart enough. Our doctor tells us all we need to know.

Wife: (entering the room) What is this? Are you flirting with my husband?

Nurse: (reexplains purpose of visit) I sure don't want to force this on you. Maybe you two will want to talk this over and let me know in a few days.

Husband: Well, maybe you could help with Johnny's temper tantrums.

Wife: Johnny's our son. Listen, don't call us, we'll call you.

Nurse: Well, I'll expect a call in 2 or 3 days. I'll check with you if I don't hear from you by then. Let's exchange phone numbers.

Husband and Wife: (in unison) Well—OK.

Although the nurse had different cultural values from those of the first family, a Spanish American family, this alone cannot explain the difficulty that she had in establishing rapport with that family. In the second family interaction, the nurse may not have fully understood the family's special biases and operating procedures, yet she was able to remain nondefensive and to pursue her goal of engaging the family in a potential working alliance.

Using the Family's Language

Besides understanding the family's cultural background and its own view of the world and way of doing things, you need to use verbal and nonverbal language that both you and the family are comfortable with. The following two segments from nurse-family interactions illustrate how important using the family's language can be for encouraging communication.

First Family

Nurse: Hiya, Dot.

Daughter (tensing up) My mother prefers to be called Mrs. Walker.

Mrs. Walker: Did you bring the necessary information, Miss Dwight?

Nurse: Oh yeah, I have it right here. Now, where the hell is it? (fumbling through her papers)

Daughter: (blushes and leaves the room) Excuse me, please.

Second Family

Nurse: Good afternoon, Mr. Newman.

Mr. Newman: Hi sweetie. You're really looking cute today.

Nurse: (clearing her throat) Umm, is you wife here? I brought the information that she requested.

Mrs. Newman: (calling from kitchen) Who's there, Charlie?

Mr. Newman: It's that cute little nurse.

Nurse: Can we sit down in the living room to discuss this?

Mrs. Newman: (calling from the kitchen) Come on in here; the coffee pot's on.

Nurse: No thanks. I'd like you to come out here and discuss this information.

In both cases, the nurse used what was comfortable for him or her and did not try to speak the family's language. Of course, it is not necessary or even advisable for you to try to become something that you're not. However, it is helpful, at least initially, to use the same or approximate degree of formality as the family uses. This can help to increase the likelihood of your being accepted by the family. It is also important for you to know and observe non-verbal cultural or family rules. For example, the members of a middle-class white American family might be impressed by your steady eye contact with them and find it a sign of sincerity and openness, while in some Spanish families, too much eye contact might be interpreted as giving the evil eye (Murray and Zentner, 1975). In the same manner, touching family members may be an important way to establish rapport in some families, while in others it may be interpreted as an affront or as an impingement on their privacy. Knowing the family's cultural practices can help you somewhat, but you will also need to observe family members as they communicate nonverbally with each other, and take your cue from them.

Encouraging Democratic Values

When working with families it is helpful to encourage democratic values. There are, of course, some cultural reasons for not encouraging shared family responsibility, democratic decision making, and equal speaking time. For example, Spanish American youngsters may not be encouraged to make decisions or to speak for themselves; encouraging them to do so might make it difficult for them to be accepted by other families and by their peers (Croddy, 1975).

In white, middle-class families, however, it is useful to encourage democratic functioning. Some aspects of this include asking family members to speak for themselves, to tell their own stories to the nurse, and not to expect others to speak for them. The nurse-family interaction below shows one way to do this.

Nurse: How did this happen, Johnny?

Mother: Oh he's always in trouble.

Nurse: What exactly happened, Johnny?

Johnny: Well, I was just trying to be buddies with the kids.

You can encourage democratic functioning and speaking out in yet another way by conveying through your words and actions that all family members have a right to give their opinions and to be listened to by others. You can state this principle but you can also demonstrate it by asking for each person's opinion and then listening to what each has to say.

Refraining from Blaming or Siding with Family Members

The quickest way to be triangled in by family members is to side with one family member. When you notice that you see one family member as a victim or as someone you need to take care of, you have taken a side, placed blame, and become triangled in, and are no longer using a systems approach. In a systems approach, all family members are viewed as perpetuating an ongoing pattern. In the two examples below, family members attempt to triangle in the nurse. In the first example, the community health nurse does take sides and sets up a situation where he or she acts as the judge of who is right. Once this position is taken, family members are more likely to attack you for being unfair and are more likely to try to manipulate you to plead their case to other family members. Once you begin to judge family members and plead for them, you have taken a role in the family and are less likely to be able to maintain some sense of objectivity about that family's system patterns.

First Family
Husband-father: What do you think, isn't my son lazy?
Nurse: Well, I wouldn't say that exactly . . .
Wife-mother: Jimmy's not lazy, just interested in other things.
Jimmy: They're always picking on me.
Nurse: I can see that they do. (to husband-father) Maybe Jimmy's involved in other things.
Husband-father: Hmph! I guess I shouldn't have expected anything different from a female.
Nurse: Sorry Mr. Warren, but I didn't say that because I'm a female.

In the second exchange, the nurse refuses to take sides. Even if you refuse to side with family members, you may be the recipient of their subtle or direct anger because you are doing something different from the way the family usually functions.

Second Family
Wife: He never listens to me. All he does is complain about how dirty it is around here.
Husband: Now that's not true, honey. I do appreciate your chocolate cake, but what about those dishes that have been in the sink for days?
Wife: (looking at the nurse) Well, which one of us is right?
Nurse: I don't think it's a question of who is right and who is wrong. Sounds like you each would like the other to listen to you more.

By taking this stance, you can provide support for each family member. Helping families to examine the consequences of their behavior rather than the intent or cause of the behavior can decrease blame fixing and increase problem solving. Examples of nonconstructive blaming comments are, "It's his fault for not taking good care of me" and "You're just trying to make me feel bad."

By suggesting that families cooperate on some level to maintain behaviors, you can help to redefine their meaning. This includes asking each family member to identify the events that led up to a particular situation. Since family members are accustomed to proceeding in a familiar and often structured way, this intervention assists them to slow down repetitive interaction and obtain a clearer view of events. Comments you might make to help families to begin to redefine the meaning of family interactions are: "Before you go on to that, it's important to hear how both your wife and daughter view what's been happening in the family" and "Although it may seem as if the main problem is Timmy, let's talk about how everyone responds when Timmy acts up." Both of these comments set the stage for an examination of how more than one person is necessary for a behavior sequence to occur and recur. You can also continue to stress that it is not important whose fault things are, but it is important to talk about how the system can be changed so that everyone is more satisfied.

Modeling Clear, Effective Communication

Although the effects of what you say and do may not be immediately visible, the families you work with will take some of their cues about how to relate from listening to and watching you. If your nonverbal communication is inconsistent with your verbal communication (e.g., smiling when angry or grimacing when saying, "OK") family members will probably be less apt to trust you and to learn that you are a reliable, concerned person.

Being clear and precise in your choice of words can give the message to families that you are direct and not interested in manipulating people or in playing games with them.

As the professional in the relationship, it is up to you to structure family discussions. Some of the areas in which you can demonstrate communication are the following:

1 Collaborating on treatment goals, e.g., "I have some ideas about how I can be helpful to you, but it is important that you tell me your ideas too."

2 Sharing perceptions about how treatment is progressing, e.g., "My impression is that we are working at cross purposes; how do you see our work together?"

3 Setting up family contracts, e.g., "I can help you to discuss family behaviors that you want to change, and to work out a system where you help one another to achieve this change."

It is not unusual for nurses to feel anxious about taking the lead in structuring family discussions. When working with one individual, you can often be helpful by merely listening and helping people to express and explore their feelings. When dealing with a group, such as a family, it is frequently more helpful for you to take a more active role in directing the focus of the discussion. It is possible to learn much from merely observing and listening to family members.

Instituting change, however, will often require that you take the lead and teach the family how to approach family decisions differently and how to use problem-solving methods.

Eliciting Alternate Strategies for Dealing with Health Problems

Nurses sometimes get stuck in the stereotype of "I am the professional, and therefore I should have all the answers." By maintaining this stance, you will perpetuate a low level of family functioning. By suggesting that family members can participate in setting treatment goals and in evaluating a plan of care, you can encourage independent and high-level functioning. Some ways of doing this are to say, "Your ideas are important, and I need everyone's input on this" and "I would like to hear some of your ideas about the kinds of ways I can help you with health care." At first, family members may look surprised when you suggest that they are responsible for their own health care and functioning. By encouraging this idea, and by listening to their ideas, families will soon learn how to work cooperatively and collaboratively with you.

Teaching Family Members How to Disagree Constructively

Families that function ineffectively often have difficulty disagreeing without attacking. When family members attack one another in your presence, you can do a number of things to intervene. First, you can rephrase what is happening, e.g., "I think Tom is disagreeing with you, but the message may be getting lost" or "It's expected that family members will disagree from time to time and it's no cause for alarm."

You may wish to obtain additional instruction and experience so that you can begin to suggest role-playing situations where family members disagree with one another without attacking each other. Expanding this intervention level requires preplanning and a well-thought out approach prior to suggesting it to a family. Satir (1964, 1975) has produced some ideas for how families can be assisted to disagree and communicate their feelings and opinions.

Teaching Family Members How to Contract with One Another

When working with families, you may find that certain family members are always remarking, "Things would be better around here if only he or she would change." In such cases, you may suggest family contracting as a method of inducing change.

For example, if mother is always complaining that son never gets to school on time, you can suggest to the mother than she make a contract with her son that he will get to school on time if she allows him to sleep late on

Saturday morning (or whatever reward the son states would induce him to change his behavior). For this method to be effective, Malouf and Alexander (1974) suggest that all family members must negotiate contracts with one another. A contract has not been made until each family member can describe what he or she will receive for keeping the contract. These rewards must be personal, individual rewards. Comments such as, "My reward will be seeing John feeling better" indicate that a contract has not been made, while comments such as, "I won't have to get notes from his teacher about how he was late again to school" indicate a personal, individual reward and a potential contract. Contracting is a technique that requires additional supervision and experience to perfect. Behavioral contracts are discussed further in Chapter 8. Chapter 12 presents a Family Observation and Intervention Guide that is meant to be a working tool for you to use in family assessment and intervention.

SUMMARY

Beginning to define yourself in your own family will help you to be a more effective practitioner with other families. The way you conduct a family interview will depend on the purpose of the interview and on your personal preferences for structure. A genogram is both an assessment and intervention tool that can give you information about multigenerational interactions and stress points as well as provide a focus for family interaction. You can encourage family communication by establishing rapport; using the family's language; encouraging democratic values; refraining from blaming or siding with family members; modeling clear, effective communication; eliciting alternative strategies for dealing with health problems; teaching family members how to disagree constructively and contract with one another.

PRACTICE EXERCISES

1 Using Figure 6-1 as a guide, construct a genogram for your own family.
2 Think of ways to use the genogram technique with a family.
3 Think of questions that you might ask during a family interview for any of the following purposes.
   a A new child has just been born.
   b A family member is about to be hospitalized.
   c The first child is starting school.
   d The first child is going away to college.
   e A parent is being hospitalized.
   f A parent is experiencing a midlife career crisis.

REVIEW

Multiple-Choice Questions

Which statements would be appropriate to ask if the purpose of the family interview is to learn about the family's attitude toward and behavior regarding health care?

a "How does Timmy deal with upsetting situations?"
b "What does each family member do for recreation?"
c "How does Timmy get along with his father?"
d "Where do family members go for help when they feel ill?"

Listing

List ways to define yourself in your own family of origin.

_____

_____

_____

Matching Terms

Match techniques for encouraging family communication with the examples by placing the correct letter in front of the appropriate technique.

Technique	Examples
1 _____ establishing rapport	**a** "What are your ideas for how to deal with this?"
2 _____ using the family's language	**b** being as formal as the family is
3 _____ encouraging democratic values	**c** asking for everyone's opinion
4 _____ eliciting alternate strategies	**d** being nondefensive and clear

REFERENCES

Bowen, M. 1975. Family therapy after twenty years. Paper distributed at the Center for Family Learning Conference, January 24, 1976, New Rochelle, New York.
_____ 1976. Toward the differentiation of self in one's family of origin. Paper distributed at the Center for Family Learning Conference, January 24, 1976, New Rochelle, New York.

Croddy, B. 1975. The therapist was a gringa. In *The psychiatric nurse as family therapist*, ed. S. Smoyak, pp. 39–45. New York: Wiley.

Ferber, A. et al. 1973. *The book of family therapy*. Boston: Houghton Mifflin.

Gosciewski, F. 1975. Using family photographs to improve communication in therapy sessions. *Hospital and Community Psychiatry* 26:641–642.

Hymovich, D. 1974. Incorporating the family into care. *Journal of the New York State Nurses Association* 5:9–14.

Malouf, R., and Alexander, J. 1974. Family crisis intervention: a model and technique of training. In *Therapeutic needs of the family*, eds. R. Hardy and J. Cull, pp. 47–55. Springfield, Ill.: Thomas.

Murray, R., and Zentner, J. 1975. *Nursing concepts for health promotion*. Englewood Cliffs, N.J.: Prentice-Hall.

Satir, V. 1964. *Conjoint family therapy*. Palo Alto: Science and Behavior Books.

_____ et al. 1975. *Helping families change*. New York: Aronson.

Sheehy, G. 1976. *Passages: predictable crises of adult life*, New York: Dutton.

Chapter 7

Substance Abuse

LEARNING OBJECTIVES

When you finish this chapter, you should be able to:

- List two current theoretical explanations for alcoholism
- List four roles to avoid when working with people who abuse alcohol
- Identify factors that influence drug abuse
- Identify interventions for people who abuse drugs
- List steps to use to teach people to reduce and maintain their weight

This chapter includes assessments and interventions where alcohol, drugs, or food is abused. Substance abuse in all of these areas seems to be no simple matter; individual, interpersonal, cultural, and legislative factors often interrelate to lead to abuse in these areas.

ALCOHOL ABUSE

Denial is a recurring theme in both those who abuse alcohol and in those who care for them. There is a tendency for physicians to refuse to recognize alcohol

abuse in adult populations (Zimberg, 1974; Twerski, 1974). Even nursing edu-
cators seem to deny the importance of substance abuse as Burkhalter (1975) has
demonstrated in her study of curriculum content in this area.

At the same time, there are strong societal pressures to condone alcohol use
as all right, and even to isolate people who refuse to have a drink for social
reasons. Bacon (1974) has found that the frequency of drunkenness increases in
societies where infants are not allowed to be dependent, where demands for
achievement in childhood are heavy, and where dependent behavior in adulthood is not tolerated. Such a description fits our achievement-oriented society,
and may explain why alcohol abuse in on the increase.

The thrust in alcohol treatment today seems to be away from viewing alcoholism as a disease or as a mental illness, and toward a view of alcohol usage as
a learned and reinforced response to depression, anxiety, and negative interpersonal relationships (Carroll, 1975; Marlatt, 1973; Finlay, 1974). Going along
with this social learning approach is the attempt to view alcoholism as a symptom of family disorganization and ineffectiveness (Berne, 1964; Ablon, 1974;
Kennedy, 1976; Steinglass, 1976).

Abuse problems with alcohol occur in people from age 8 to age 75, and at
all socioeconomic levels. Teenage drinking is increasing, and a report of a 1975
survey from the National Institute on Alcohol Abuse and Alcoholism disclosed
that one child in every four at age 13 or younger drinks frequently enough and
in sufficient quantities to be classified as a moderate drinker. Parental drinking
is related to their children's drinking; parents who drink are twice as likely to
have adolescents who drink than are nondrinking parents (Horoshak, 1976).

In the adult population there are 10 million identified alcoholics (Hendrickson, 1975) and it is not clear how many alcholics have not been identified due
to denial on their part or on that of their caregivers. Zimberg (1974) reported
alcohol abuse is a serious problem in urban and suburban people 65- to 74-
years-old and especially in elderly widowers.

Assessing Alcoholism

Each major age grouping (adolescent, adult, and geriatric) has special problems
in assessment. In addition, the point at which you come in contact with a person
who has a drinking problem will influence your assessment. For example,
Heinemann and Estes (1976) have noted that a person's acceptance of the
diagnosis of alcoholism comes in phases that are similar to that of the grief
process (see Chapter 4). People who are in the denial phase of alcoholism will
present special problems in assessment.

Horoshak (1976) suggests that rapport be established on some level with
adolescent drinkers prior to discussing their drinking patterns. Once this rapport
has been established, you can begin to ask teenagers to talk about themselves.
Once you have gained their confidence, you will be able to comment on their
difficulty in relating to others by asking a question such as, "It seems you might

have a problem there—how do you usually handle it?" If the answer is that they handle it by getting drunk, that is your cue to suggest a counseling group with other teenagers who are going through "the same things you are." You must, of course, be aware of a suitable counseling group and/or start one yourself with supervision from a more experienced group leader.

In assessing the adult alcoholic, obvious physical clues are flushed face, blood-shot or puffy eyes, trembling or sweaty heands, protruding abdomen, excessively dry skin, and dilated blood vessels on the face. Less obvious signs include rest-lessness, irritability, fatigue, frequent GI upsets, colds, a pattern of Friday and Monday absences from work, an elevation in blood pressure and pulse, decreased vision, burn marks on fingers (due to nerve damage), muscular cramps (especially in the calf area), and complaints of nausea and vomiting (Hendrickson, 1975). Sleep disturbances and a deteriorating sex life are other complaints associated with alcoholism (Heinemann and Estes, 1976).

In assessing the person over 65, Zimberg (1974) distinguishes between those who have been abusing alcohol for months or years, and those who started to drink as a reaction to the stress of aging. In the first group, Zimberg found that drinking was a reaction to loneliness and depression. In the second group, alcohol may be used relatively recently as a way to deal with the stress of aging or with the recent loss of a spouse. For these reasons it is important to determine whether drinking is being used to deal with an underlying lifelong depressive style or whether it is a grief reaction to a recent loss. You can ask clients if and when they began to experience loss of appetite and difficulty sleeping. Since alcohol is a depressant, and since the elderly may be less tolerant of its effects than younger people are, it would seem to be counterindicated as a prescription or intervention for relaxation with this population.

Because people who drink a lot are "notorious for being inaccurate histor-ians" (Heinemann and Estes, 1976) they should be asked questions for the purpose of eliciting descriptions.

- What symptoms have you had recently?
- What kinds of alcoholic beverages do you drink?
- What other drugs are you taking?
- Who can you talk to about your problems?
- What is your usual eating pattern?
- What reactions do you have after you stop drinking?
- Where do you do your drinking? With whom?
- What changes have there been in your life recently?
- When you drink, do you ever lose track of time or forget what happened the night before?
- When was the last time you missed work (social engagements)?
- What does drinking do for you?
- When do you find yourself reaching for a drink?
- What effect has drinking had on your job (family life, social life, hobbies)?

Many people will not reply candidly to this type of questioning, but how they respond or what they omit or how they evade certain facts can also be clues to their use of alcohol. Family members, clergy, and family physicians may provide you with further data for assessment. Asking people why they drink is usually futile since they often do not know why, and will probably invent reasons. Pretending that alcohol is not a problem only reinforces denial.

The Alcoholic Game

Berne (1964) was one of the first to examine alcoholism as an interpersonal situation. He referred to alcoholism as a life game where the major roles are It (the alcoholic), Persecutor, Patsy, Connection, and Rescuer. A number of roles may be played by the alcoholic person and/or spouse; at various times the person with the drinking problem may berate him- or herself and become *Persecutor* or evoke derogatory remarks from the spouse or from you. *Rescuer* is often played by a nurse or doctor who wants to take care of others. Rescuer is the role the reformed alcoholic plays in Alcoholics Anonymous. *Patsy* is the person who supplies money, alcohol, or sympathy for the drinker. *Connection* is the direct source of supply of alcohol.

In the initial stages of this game the spouse may play Patsy by undressing the other and by making coffee for him or her. In the morning both spouses may take turns playing Persecutor ("How can you do this to me?" or "How can you let me do this to myself?") According to Berne, the game is maintained because it affords the drinker an opportunity to provoke others into taking care of and then forgiving him or her without allowing intimacy to develop between the participants. The roles of Rescuer and Persecutor are satisfying in some ways to people who wish to take care of others. Because you are in a role where patients or clients may try to get you to care for them, you are in a prime position to be cast in these roles.

Another role you may find easy to play is that of Patsy. The person who drinks may try to manipulate you by telling you something like, "I like you better than other people" or "I can really talk to you" or "You're the only one I trust." By depending on you to keep him or her away from drinking the alcoholic may become quite angry if drinking should recur, and may blame you for failing to stop its recurrence.

You can avoid these roles by declining to play the game. Instead, you might collaborate with the client to work toward goals and to find out what is disturbing him or her. Also, by trying to place the person's behavior within a game structure, it is much easier not to get into a win-lose situation. Since the game is to change rules at will and then be punished and then be forgiven for the infraction, it is important to maintain matter-of-fact consistency about rules and agreed-upon goals. Some questions that you can ask to assess your own game playing are:

- Do I feel angry when the person relapses into drinking? (Persecutor role)
- Do I feel that only I can help this person? (Rescuer role)
- Do I change rules or goals at the whim of clients? (Patsy role)
- Do I feel guilty when clients attack me for not helping them to stop drinking? (Patsy role)

Some questions that you can ask to assess the roles family members are playing are:

- Does the spouse or child of the drinker conceal his or her drinking habits? (Patsy role)
- Does the spouse or child refuse any assistance and claim that only he or she can help the drinker? (Rescuer role)
- Does the spouse or child denigrate the drinker to you or berate the drinker to his or her face? (Persecutor role)
- Does the spouse buy or provide alcohol for the drinker? (Connection role)
- Does the spouse or child take care of the drinker as if he or she were the child? (Rescuer role)

Intervention

It is only at the point where the person who abuses alcohol can see benefits from relating with others and can see life experiences as rewarding that he or she will give up drinking. Therefore, although you can offer a relationship and alternatives in terms of treatment programs and life experiences, it is the individual who must decide to give up the game. Giving up the game necessitates examining the underlying problems of anxiety, depression, and loneliness.

For teenagers, important scenes (such as the youth who comes home drunk) can be played out at group sessions and used as starting points for discussing anxiety, anger, and depression and how to deal with these feelings in constructive ways. It is also important for you, as a nurse, not to become embroiled in the family's game where the parents of the teenager seem to you to have rejected their child; if you do this, you have accepted the role of Rescuer.

Role-playing situations can be used with adults also. Assertiveness training where people are taught to speak up for their rights as individuals (Martorano, 1973) and desensitization training where people learn to control their anxiety in social situations (Pucel, 1972) also show promise as treatment modalities.

Ditzler (1976) suggests that people who abuse alcohol should be treated with a present-oriented approach. People should be encouraged to express their anger and anxiety over current situations. Ditzler also discusses the importance of realizing that sympathy, support, and prompt relief of physical and emotional pain may not be the most useful approach. Suggesting that pain-killing medications or other types of drugs can help the person who abuses alcohol merely reinforces in him or her the idea that life problems can be cured by a magic pill. People can and should be encouraged to search for alternate ways to deal with their discomfort. You will help your clients in this endeavor by realizing that a certain amount of anxiety is necessary to encourage problem solving and behavioral change.

For members of the geriatric population, carefully monitored antidepressant medication and one-to-one counseling may be most helpful. Zimberg (1974) cautions against the use of wine or liquor in nursing homes, hospitals, or the home because depression may increase as a result and even small amounts of alcohol may have strong effects on the imbiber due to the increased sensitivity that age brings.

Prevention

There are a number of ways in which you can act to prevent the difficulties associated with alcohol abuse. One way is to provide parents and students with alcohol-related problems with instructional materials and to help develop organized learning experiences for them. Some sources of information in this area appear at the end of the chapter reference section.

Another way to prevent later drinking difficulties is to identify early signs of preadolescent drinking. Zucker (1976) suggests that youngsters between the ages of 11 and 14 can be reached more easily than older teenagers because adolescent peer-interaction patterns have not yet solidified. He found a strong relationship between problem drinking among adolescents and serious physical aggression, early and frequent sexual experiences, and parental defiance. Zucker suggests that a direct information-gathering program be used to detect alcohol abuse. The school is the obvious place for such a program. Youngsters who are depressed or anxious about themselves or their drinking behavior may be responsive to questionnaires or surveys. Other students with the potential of becoming alcohol abusers can be screened for characteristics such as low grades, lack of involvement in school activities, and greater knowledge of delinquent and drug culture slang. These youngsters can be given peer group projects that meet the real needs of the school or community and that provide them with a supervised and constructive outlet for their energy.

DRUG ABUSE

Denial is also a recurring theme in conjunction with drug abuse. Cousins (1976) points out that, on one hand, our society is indignant at people who abuse drugs and that, on the other hand, it is seemingly oblivious to the everyday misuse of prescription drugs.

Is no moral or legal issue posed by the fact that some doctors make hundreds of thousands of dollars a year out of drug-dependent indigents? And what about pharmacies, which are doing a land-office business in dangerous drugs, with the state as sponsor and underwriter?

Despite the questions that Cousins raises, nurses (Brink, 1973) and the general public (Cant, 1976) continue to cast drug abusers in the bad person role and to vacillate between feeling angry (Persecutor role) and acting motherly (Rescuer role) when dealing with people who have been identified as drug addicts.

Yet the problem is even larger. There is a known correlation between abuse of legal drugs and suicide attempts (DuPont, 1976), a growing feeling that Ritalin may be being misused in schools as a treatment for hyperactivity (Bosco, 1975; Witter, 1971), and the charge that even our legal monitoring agencies are lax (FDA accused of laxity, *New York Times,* July 25, 1976).

Given the degree of denial that exists in our society that allows heroin addiction to be regarded as bad and self-prescription or overindulgence in drugs such as Valium or Librium as OK, it is difficult to determine exactly what it is that leads to drug abuse. One prominent theory is that addiction is a way of surviving, of avoiding painful life experiences. To Ottenberg (1974, p.19) "Addiction gives meaning and purpose to an addict's life; only through substituting other values can a cure occur." Another theory is that boredom and peer influence lead to drug abuse (Warner, 1973). A more recent theory is that drug abuse, especially in adolescence, is a symptom of family disorganization and ineffective communication. Huberty (1975) found that if the family of adolescent drug abusers was not included in treatment, interventions were doomed to fail. In the families he studied, he found that there was a tendency to deny or be ignorant of the effects of the drug being abused, a failure to accept responsibility, an inability to communicate thoughts and feelings openly, and evidences of parental drug abuse.

Randell (1971), too, takes a family-oriented approach to drug abuse. He views adolescence as a crisis period during which the adolescent is struggling to break away from the dependent behaviors of childhood and in which there is an inconsistency between the expectations of the adolescent and those of his or her parents as well as inconsistencies that the adolescent encounters in the real world. One way that adolescents may resolve this crisis is by starting to use drugs and in them finding a relief for the internal and external growth pressures that he or she is feeling.

Interventions

The first intervention you can make when dealing with people who abuse drugs it to examine your own biases and reactions. Some questions to ask yourself in this regard are:

- Do I view the abuse of some drugs (such as nicotine, caffeine, or alcohol) as more acceptable than the abuse of others?
- Do I feel in conflict about persecuting versus rescuing people who abuse drugs?

• Do I expect the client to abstain completely from drugs rather than accept his or her partial abstinence or movement toward abstinence?

• Do I see drug abuse as an individual problem or as the result of complex factors?

Once you have sorted out your thoughts and feelings about drug abuse, you can begin to be helpful to people who abuse drugs. Further interventions can be divided into three categories: individual and group, family, and educational efforts.

Warner (1973) suggests that the best way to teach people who abuse drugs how to be independent and to solve their problems is to engage them in a collaborative approach to treatment goals. She thinks that, although people who abuse drugs may make many demands to be cared for, setting limits, being consistent, and assisting people to work through their crises by examining the pros and cons of their behavior, and then helping them to act on their own decisions is the most helpful course. Warner described waiting until her client, Karen, was ready to proceed with getting a driver's license as a crucial step in timing her interventions with this person. The client had been driving illegally until then, partially due to her fears that she would fail the examination. When her client was ready, the nurse accompanied her to the testing center where Karen passed her test and subsequently increased her self-esteem.

Other strategies to use with drug abusers who have withdrawn into themselves is to provide them with sensory input, to start rap groups where provocative discussions may draw them out, and to use video- or audiotape playback to stimulate interaction among them (Dambacher, 1971).

Family interventions would include teaching family members how to communicate more openly and directly with one another. Klimenko (1968) suggests using comments such as, "Tell that to your father, Lloyd" and "You let her get away with that?" Working with groups of families each of which has one or more members who abuse drugs can have many advantages. Klimenko suggests that co-leaders can serve as role models to teach family members how to work collaboratively and disagree constructively with each other. Being a leader of a family group requires additional instruction and supervision and should not be attempted prior to obtaining this experience.

If family members cannot participate in family or group sessions, you may give them specific directions to follow at home as a way of learning how to communicate with one another. For example, you might suggest that they plan the family food list and go shopping together, or plan a day excursion and see it through. Children can be asked to spend a weekend with their parents and to try to get to know them as people. A less demanding task would be for the family to have one full meal together without letting TV, radio, or newspapers hinder communication. It is surprising how in many families communication between members is prevented by such physical barriers as not being in the same room facing one another, or hiding behind the evening newspaper or in front of the TV. You can suggest that family members discuss their ideas with one another and decide on other things they can do together.

Prevention

One of the easiest ways to turn off potential drug users is to preach to them about the evils of drug abuse (Bard, 1975). One way to convey your interest in understanding the drug abuser's views is to tell him that you want to learn about his experiences. Parents could be encouraged to ask their children about the positive aspects of drugs rather than to lecture them on the negative ones (Weil, 1972).

Warner (1973) reviewed the research on preventive drug abuse programs and found that antidrug attitudes among college students were promoted more by focusing on values and attitudes than on providing information about drugs. Simon et al. (1972) have compiled practical strategies for teachers and students in the values clarification area. Most of these exercises could be modified and used by you with drug abusers and/or their families. The values clarification approach teaches people to sort out their thoughts and feelings, to become aware of what they value, to choose from a set of alternative beliefs and behaviors, and then to act on those choices with consistency.

There are other areas in which you can practice preventive intervention. You can reduce drug-taking errors, self-medication, and you can assist clients in defining alternate actions other than the taking of medication in order to cope with problems of living. A study by Hulka (1976) found that of all the errors in medication usage, combined physician and patient errors totaled 58 percent. Although physicians labelled these patients noncompliant, the researchers found that the major problem was lack of communication. Patients did not know what was expected of them in relation to drug taking, and did not know the function of the drugs that they were taking. This type of helper-helpee relationship would seem to promote the under- and overusage of drugs. As a nurse, you can stem this tide by making sure that each person you work with knows the medications that he or she is taking and the function of each one. You can also discourage self-medication through the use of prescribed and over-the-counter drugs. As more and more drugs (including aspirin) come under fire for being more harmful than helpful (Cousins, 1975), it behooves you, as a nurse, to encourage your clients to use alternate measures for dealing with health problems. For example, there are many nursing interventions beside pain medication that can be used to relieve pain (Clark, 1977).

FOOD ABUSE

Every year more than 25 million Americans attempt to take off excess weight and keep it off (Robbins and Fisher, 1976). Some are successful; others are not.

Success or failure is probably related to early, learned, family experiences. The roots of obesity are beginning to be traced back to infant feeding behaviors where rapid weight gain and proliferation of fat cells occur. Bottle-fed babies seem to have a higher potential for obesity than breastfed babies because they tend to show more rapid weight gain. Current research by Crow (1976) is attempting to examine how infants regulate their own food intake, what role early learning may play in the amount of milk the infant drinks, and whether different ways of providing food influence the infant's intake. Garn (1976) has also emphasized the importance of learning in obesity. He has found that the children of obese parents are several times fatter than the children of lean parents. He discounts heredity as an explanation, and concludes that attitudes toward food, eating, and exercise are learned in the family and reinforced in the home. There are other results that indicate that learning plays a large role in obesity. For example, obese people eat whenever they think it is time to eat and are less influenced by actual time than are thinner people, and obese people are more influenced by the taste of food than others are (Hartie, 1975).

It would seem that much overeating is due to faulty feedback from hunger control mechanisms and that this faulty feedback is learned. Many obese people seem unaware of how much they eat, frequently claim they never eat, yet are surprised at how much they do eat when asked to keep a record of their food intake (Hartie, 1975).

Thus, there is strong evidence that environmental cues determine overeating, and therefore it is futile to ask the obese peron to exert self-control. Since weight gain is not noticeable until much later than the ingestion of food, it is necessary to rearrange the eating environment so as to reduce eating behavior. If the pattern of eating is not changed, obese people will reduce and then gain back all the weight that was lost.

A treatment approach that shows promise in weight reduction and maintenance is *behavior therapy* or *behavior modification*. The focus of attention in this approach is on the observable behavior associated with weight loss. You can play a major part in the treatment of obesity. This is a natural role for you since you come into contact with overweight people in the hospital and community far more than members of other disciplines do. However, if you expect that merely instructing clients in the proper diet will result in weight reduction and maintenance, you will probably be quite frustrated.

Food Intake and Environment Record

The first step in a weight reduction program is for you and the client to become aware of the client's eating patterns. These patterns should be recorded and should include the following elements:

- Type, quantity, and caloric value of foods eaten
- Where food is eaten

- When food is eaten
- Social responses to eating

The client can be told to purchase a notebook that he or she is to carry at all times and use to record eating data. Table 7-1 shows one way to record this information. Note how many different places the client eats in, how he overlooks the danish and beer, how quickly most food is eaten, and how many other social activities are occurring at the time he is eating. During this baseline or data-collection phase, tell the client not to diet or try to reduce.

An initial weight reduction often occurs at this point when people begin to realize what they are eating, and begin spending more time recording, thus leaving less time for eating. Go over the food record with the client, praising his or her attempts to remember what was eaten, but *never* chide the client for what was eaten. This record should be kept for several weeks so that patterns in eating can be identified. You may decide whether you wish to have the client record

Table 7-1 My Eating Patterns: One Client's Eating Pattern for One Day

What I ate and drank	Where I ate and drank it	When I ate and drank it	How I ate and drank it	What else was I doing while I was eating
2 Oreo cookies	Living room	8:00 p.m.	Quickly	Watching TV
Small bag potato chips	Living room	10:00 p.m.	Quickly with a beer	Watching TV
Black coffee	Office desk	9:30 a.m.	With a danish	Talking to secretary
Hamburger (without bun), cottage cheese, black coffee	Lunch room	Noon	In a hurry	Talking with friends
Almond Joy	Office hallway	1:30 p.m.	On way to desk	
Coke	Office desk	3:00 p.m.	During work breaks	Working puzzle
Salad, low-calorie dressing, chicken breast, creamed corn, french fries, 2 slices bread	Dining room table	6:00 p.m.	In company of family	Arguing about where to go on vacation

caloric values or not; if the client feels guilty (and most do) it may be best not to include this exercise at first.

Other Initial Procedures

You may wish to ask clients to purchase graph paper and chart their weight every day. This directive requires that they weigh themselves daily. It is important that you tell them to do so at the same time every day (Robbins and Fisher, 1976).

Another technique that you may use is to ask them to visualize how they wish to look in the future. You might say, "Picture your slim, trim self." It is important that you help clients to identify realistic goals to work toward, e.g., a weight reduction of 5 or 10 pounds. Once this goal has been reached, another can be set. Goals that can be reached in relatively short periods of time will provide stronger motivation than goals that require several months or a year to reach.

Clients should be told to begin an excercise program after they have had a physical examination. They can also place reminders to themselves in strategic areas. For example, pictures of their real or ideal self, or notes such as "Don't open this door!" can be pasted on the refrigerator door. Clients can also be directed to make a list of activities that they enjoy that have nothing to do with eating; these may include hobbies, recreational activities, and so on.

Weight Reduction Techniques

Once both you and the client know his or her pattern of eating, you can begin to help the client structure a different eating environment for him- or herself. Hartie (1975) and Robbins and Fisher (1976) suggest some guidelines. The following ones are an adaptation and combination of their suggestions.

Make It Difficult to Overeat
Never go shopping when you are hungry.
Only buy foods that require preparation.
Only prepare enough food to serve a small portion.
Use small plates.
Force yourself to eat slowly.
Put your fork or spoon down between each bite.
Use chopsticks if possible.
Chew each mouthful at least twenty times.
Drink at least one glass of water with each meal.

Work to Reduce the Number of Times Per Day That You Eat
Each time you eat one more time than your limit, punish yourself in some small, nondangerous way, e.g., by not allowing yourself to wear a favorite

article of clothing, or by forcing yourself to watch a TV program that you hate, or by writing down a list of reasons why you should not eat.

Reward yourself by doing one of your favorite activities when you stick to your goal.

Work to Decrease the Number of Areas Where You Eat

Stay out of eating areas unless you plan to eat.

Eat in only one location in your chosen place(s), e.g., only when sitting at the table.

Never eat standing up.

Make Eating Time Only for Eating

Turn off the TV and radio.

Do not read or talk when eating.

Concentrate only on chewing the food that you are eating.

Leave the table when you have finished eating.

Increase Your Energy Output

Park your car several blocks from where you work.

Get off the elevator one flight from where you are going and walk the last flight.

Every time you get an urge to eat, take a walk down the hall or outside the building, or do a simple exercise.

Prevention

Keep up with the newest research on bottle versus breatfeeding in terms of which produces more fat cells. Counsel mothers of infants and obese parents about how their children learn eating habits. Try to convince obese parents to begin behavioral modification methods to decrease their weight; if they comply, their children will benefit by learning healthier eating habits. Form support and/or behavior modification nutrition groups for overweight people.

SUMMARY

Denial is a recurring theme in both those who abuse alcohol and in those who care for them. Treatment of alcoholism is moving away from a disease approach and toward a view of alcohol as a learned response to depression, anxiety, negative interpersonal relationships, and family disorganization. Assessments differ by age group. Being able to identify alcoholic game roles can be helpful in not taking roles in the game. You can prevent alcohol abuse by providing instructional materials, by identifying early signs of preadolescent drinking, and by working with peer groups and families to find alternate ways to deal with their feelings.

Our society shows denial in its permissive attitude toward the abuse of legal drugs and in its overreaction to the abuse of illegal drugs. Drug abuse, too, is currently being seen as a symptom of family disorganization, as an inability to communicate with others, and as a perceived solution to developmental crises. Collaborative approaches with clients who abuse drugs and use of appropriate timing, rap groups, and audiovisual methods can help you to reach people who abuse drugs. Values clarification seems more useful than preaching about the evils of drugs.

Food abuse seems to be a learned response that can be unlearned through the change of environmental cues. The use of behavior modification techniques such as intake records and environmental structuring holds promise for weight reduction and maintenance.

When you work with any abuse problem, it is vitally important that you examine your own biases toward and reactions to people who have these problems.

PRACTICE EXERCISES

1 Talk with family members in a family where one member abuses alcohol. Try to figure out what role(s) each plays in the game.
2 Pick one age grouping or substance abuse grouping. Plan, and then carry out, one intervention for one client or family.
3 Pick one age grouping or substance abuse grouping. Plan, and then carry out, one preventive action for one client, group, or family.

REVIEW

Multiple-Choice Questions

1 Which of the following factors increase drug abuse?
  a Legal and medical authority to use legal drugs.
  b Decrease in suicide attempts.
  c Decreased hyperactivity in school children.
  d Boredom, peer influence, family disorganization.
2 Which of the following interventions seem most helpful for people who abuse drugs?
  a Helpers are in touch with their own biases.
  b Helpers predefine a treatment program.
  c Family members are taught how to communicate more openly and directly with one another.
  d Information about types of drugs and their effects is freely given.
  e Each client is told the name, action, side effects, and purpose of each prescribed drug.

Listing

1 List two current theoretical explanations for alcoholism.

_____

_____

2 List four roles to avoid when working with people who abuse alcohol.

_____

3 List steps to use to teach people to reduce and maintain their weight.

_____

_____

_____

REFERENCES

Ablon, A. 1974. Al-Anon family groups. *American Journal of Psychotherapy* 29:30–45.

Bard, B. 1975. The failure of our school drug abuse programs. *Phi Delta Kappan* 57, 4:251–255.

Bacon, M. 1974. Dependency-conflict hypothesis and the frequency of drunkenness. *Quarterly Journal of Studies on Alcohol* 35, 3:863–875.

Berne, E. 1964. *Games people play.* New York: Grove.

Bosco, J. 1975. Behavior modification drugs and the schools: the case of ritalin. *Phi Delta Kappan* 57, 7:489–492.

Brink, P. 1973. Nurses' attitude toward heroin addicts. *Journal of Psychiatric Nursing* 11, 2:7–12.

Bruch, H. 1973. *Eating disorders: obesity, anorexia nervosa, and the person within.* New York: Basic Books.

Burkhalter, P. 1975. Alcoholism, drug abuse and drug addiction: a study of nursing education. *Journal of Nursing Education* 14, 2:30–36.

Cant, G. 1976. Valiumania. *New York Times Magazine* February 1, pp. 34–44.

Carroll, J. 1975. "Mental illness" and "disease": outmoded concepts in alcohol and drug rehabilitation. *Community Mental Health Journal* 11:418–429.

Clark, C. 1977. Pain assessment and intervention. *Nursing Concepts and Processes.* Albany: Delmar.

Cousins, N. 1975. Pain, panic and pills. *Saturday Review* May 31, pp. 4–5.

_____ 1976. Philadelphia story. *Saturday Review* October 30, p. 4.

Crow, R., and Wright, P. 1976. The development of feeding behavior in early infancy. *Nursing Mirror* 142, (April 1):57–59.

Dambacher, B., and Hellwig, K. 1971. Nursing strategies for young drug users. *Perspectives in Psychiatric Care* 9, 5:101–105.

Ditzler, J. 1976. Rehabilitation for alcoholics. *American Journal of Nursing* 76, 11:1772–1775.

DuPont, R. 1976. Psychic effects, suicide attempts cited as leading reasons for drug abuse. *Behavior Today* 7, 30:4.

Dy, A. et al. 1975. The nurse in the methadone maintenance program: expansions and transitions in role. *Journal of Psychiatric Nursing* 13, 3:17–20.

FDA accused of laxity. 1976. *New York Times* July 25.

Finlay, D. 1974. Alcoholism: illness or problem in interaction. *Social Work* 19, 4:398–405.

Flack, R., and Grayer, E. 1975. A consciousness-raising group for obese women. *Social Work* 20, 6:484–487.

Freed, E. 1973. Abstinence for alcoholics reconsidered. *Journal of Alcoholism* 8, 3:106–110.

Garn, S. 1976. Trends in fatness and the origin of obesity. *Pediatrics* 57, 4:443–456.

Hartie, A. 1975. Obesity: environmental control of eating. *Nursing Mirror* 141, (December 11):47–49.

Heinemann, E., and Estes, N. 1976. Assessing alcoholic patients. *American Journal of Nursing* 76, 5:786–789.

Hendrickson, J. 1975. The alcoholic employee: how the nurse can help. *Nursing '75* 5, (December):46–50.

Horoshak, I. 1976. Teen-age drinking: a growing problem or a problem of growing? *RN* 39, (March):63–69.

Huberty, D. 1975. Treating the adolescent drug abuser: a family affair. *Contemporary Drug Problems* 4, 2:179–194.

Hulka, B. et al. 1976. Communication, compliance and concordance between physicians and patients with prescribed medications. *American Journal of Public Health* 66, 9:847–853.

Kennedy, D. 1976. Behavior of alcoholics and spouses in a simulation game situation. *Journal of Nervous and Mental Diseases* 162, 1:23–34.

Klimenko, A. 1968. Multifamily therapy in the rehabilitation of drug addicts. *Perspectives in Psychiatric Care* 6, 5:220–223.

Loxsom, R. 1975. Changing obesity patterns. *Nursing Outlook* 23, 11:711–713.

Mahoney, M. 1976. Fight fat with behavior control. *Psychology Today* 9, (May):39–41.

Marlatt, G. 1973. Learning alcoholism. *Behavior Today* 4, 43:2, 4.

Millsap, M. 1972. Occupational health nursing in an alcohol addiction program. *Nursing Clinics of North America* 7, 1:121–132.

Martorano, R. 1973. The effects of assertive and nonassertive training on alcohol consumption, mood, and socialization in chronic alcoholism. Ph.D. dissertation, Rutgers University, Newark, N.J.

Ottenberg, D. 1974. Addiction as metaphor. *Alcohol Health and Research World* (Fall): 18–20.

Pucel, J. 1972. Systematic desensitization and the reduction of social anxiety: the efficacy of using such a treatment technique as part of an alcoholic treatment program. Ph.D. dissertation, University of Missouri, Columbia, Mo.

Randell, B. 1971. Short-term group therapy with the adolescent drug offender. *Perspectives in Psychiatric Care* 9, 3:123–128.

Robbins, J., and Fisher, D. 1976. *Behavior modification: how to make and break habits.* New York: Dell.

Simon, S. et al. 1972. *Values clarification.* New York: Hart.

Steinglass, P. 1976. Experimenting with family treatment approaches to alcoholism, 1950–1975: a review. *Family Process* 15, 1:97–123.

Thorn, M., and Boudewyns, P. 1976. A behaviorally-oriented weight loss program for counseling centers. *Journal of Counseling Psychology* 23, 1:81–82.

Twerski, A. 1974. When to hospitalize the alcoholic. *Nursing Digest* 2, 2:15–22.

Walker, L. 1974. Crises of change: a case study of a heroin dependent patient. *Perspectives in Psychiatric Care* 12, 1:20–25.

Warner, R. 1973. Preventing drug abuse: where are we? *Nursing Digest* 1, 7:21–27.

Weil, A. 1972. *The natural mind: a new way of looking at the higher consciousness.* Boston: Houghton Mifflin.

Witter, C. 1971. Drugging and schooling. *Transaction* 8, 9–10:31–34.

Zimberg, S. 1974. The elderly alcoholic. *Gerontologist* 14, 3:221–224.

Zucker, R. 1976. Deviant youth should be target of prevention during ages 11–14. *NICAAA Information and Feature Service* DHEW Public. No. (ADM) 76-151, July 2.

SOURCES OF INSTRUCTIONAL MATERIALS ON ALCOHOL-RELATED PROBLEMS

National Institute on Alcohol Abuse and Alcoholism (NIAAA)

Formulates policies and goals regarding the prevention, control, and treatment of alcohol abuse. Awards grants to agencies and organizations.
Write: NIAAA, 5600 Fishers Lane, Rockville, MD 20852.

National Clearinghouse for Alcohol Information (NCALI)

Provides information, news, and pamphlets on alcohol abuse. Can provide posters, films, and research abstracts.
Write: NCALI, PO box 2345, Rockville, MD 20852.

National Council on Alcoholism (NCA)

Provides programs of public education, treatment, and community education.
Write: NCA, 2 Park Avenue, New York, NY 10016.

Alcoholics Anonymous (AA)

Self-help group that provides treatment for and free information about alcoholism. Check the listing in your local telephone book.
Write: Alcoholics Anonymous, PO Box 459, Grand Central Station, New York, NY 10017.

Al-Anon/Alateen

Self-help family groups whose purpose is to help relatives and family members to cope with the problems related to living with alcoholics.
Write: Al-Anon or Alateen, PO Box 182, Madison Square Station, New York, NY 10010.

Chapter 8

Social Learning

LEARNING OBJECTIVES

When you finish this chapter you should be able to:

- Identify behaviors that can be counted
- Identify social learning techniques

Since the family is a system of interlocking, reciprocal behaviors, family members can be taught to change their responses to others by rewarding the desired behaviors of others and thus producing family change.

THE SOCIAL LEARNING MODEL

The social learning or behavioral approach focuses on specific, observable behaviors. This approach is not primarily concerned with insight or with whether people understand why they act as they do, but rather with decreasing unsatisfying or disruptive behavior and with increasing satisfying, goal-directed behavior. As a community health nurse you will come in contact with clients who seem unmotivated. A more useful way to view this seeming noncompliance is as faulty learning. Once this view is taken, specific behaviors can be identified and counted (baseline data), and then health behavior can be reinforced.

Since human behavior is learned, it can also be unlearned. You may wish to use the behavioral or social learning model with individual clients and families, or with yourself or to teach your colleagues how to make constructive habits or break nonconstructive ones.

The idea of deliberately manipulating a learning environment seems to run counter to the idea of encouraging independent action. Yet, parents, teachers, and even nurses use some principles of learning theory whenever they praise behavior that they think is acceptable, or punish or ignore behaviors that they find unacceptable. The behavioral approach is merely a systematic way to reward more satisfying behaviors and to not reward disruptive or unsatisfying behaviors. Particularly with adults, but even with children, you cannot use these techniques unless the client plays a role in determining the direction of his or her own behavior change. Clients can participate in such techniques by making decisions about what behavior is to be changed, by studying their own behavior in the pretreatment phase, and by choosing the consequences or reinforcers (rewards or punishments) for various behaviors. By including clients as active participants in decision making you can reduce ethical problems concerned with manipulating the learning environment (Carignan, 1974).

STEPS IN TEACHING MORE EFFECTIVE BEHAVIOR

The first step in learning more effective behavior is to identify the behavior to be changed. Behavior is an action (Berni and Fordyce, 1973), not a feeling, attitude, or mood. Behaviors must be pinpointed and expressed in such a way that they can be counted. Table 8-1 shows examples of behaviors that can and cannot be counted.

Once the behavior is expressed in countable terms, you and/or the client can begin to gather baseline data. This data is information gathered prior to treatment; the pinpointed behavior is counted or measured to see how often it occurs now. This data can be charted and hung in the client's home or in the nurse's office or it can be recorded on the treatment chart. Data from this "before" or baseline phase can be used later to check progress toward the goal. There are a number of ways to count behavior: frequency, rate over time, or how long the behavior continues. The method used to count depends on the behavior. For example, you may use the frequency method to count arguments with the nurse, the rate over time method to measure weight gain or loss, and the duration method to measure how long the client sits up in a chair. A notebook, graph, or chart can be used to gather baseline data.

Table 8-1 Examples of Behaviors That Can and Cannot Be Counted

Countable behaviors	General behaviors or internal states
Making bed	Being neat
Washing dishes	Being motivated
Not scattering underwear on floor	Being resistant
Walking down hall	Being depressed
Calling for help	Being angry
Brushing teeth	Being negative
Taking medication	Losing your memory
Arguing with nurse	Regressing
Drinking fluids	Increasing your mobility
Using the commode	Being afraid
Losing weight	Being active
Gaining weight	Feeling guilty
Joining group activities	Being noncompliant
Biting your nails	Being happy
Smoking a cigarette	Grieving
Forgetting people's names	Being hostile
Being on time for work	Increasing your social relationships
Finishing reports	Improving your communication

Figure 8-1 shows baseline data for self-feeding, being late to work, and gaining weight.

The next step in decreasing undesirable or increasing desirable behavior is to find out what is rewarding and punishing to the particular client. Table 8-2 shows reinforcers for one nurse who was chronically late to work. Clients, too, can be asked to make such a list. There are some nearly universal rewards such as attention, smiles, praise, and candy or other sweets. In situations where the client is uncooperative and refuses to tell you what is rewarding you can ask family members what is pleasing to the client, read the chart for hints, or use a universal reward. Of course, giving sweets to someone with diabetes or who wants to lose weight would be self-defeating. You also cannot use a reward if you cannot establish control over when the reinforcer

Table 8-2 Reinforcers for One Nurse

Positive, rewarding reinforcers	Negative, punishing reinforcers
Eating ice cream	Watching cartoons
Seeing a movie	Working overtime
Sleeping late on weekends	Being reminded that I'm late
Talking with other nurses	Doing dishes
Going dancing	Doing reports
Reading mysteries	Eating cottage cheese

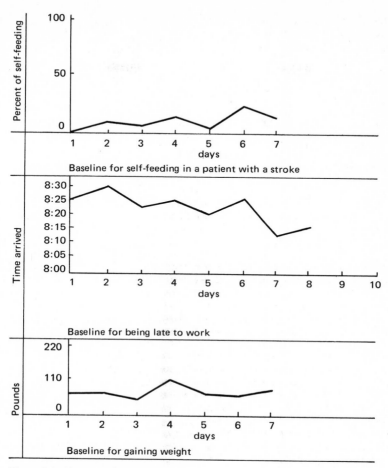

Figure 8-1 Examples of baseline data.

is dispensed. For example, if a family lets a child watch TV whether she has completed her homework or not, watching TV cannot be used as a reward for the child's doing her homework. Because you can control relatively few rewards, it is wise to enlist the aid of families, school personnel, and whomever it is who dispenses rewards. The best way to do this is to reward them for helping you by giving them attention, by not scolding them when they do not comply, and by using whatever other things that you notice are rewarding to them.

In order to increase the occurrence of a goal-directed behavior, the reward must immediately follow movement toward that behavior. Giving the client an ice cream cone two days after he or she walked around the block will not increase the walking behavior.

In some cases it may be unrealistic or impossible to provide the reinforcer immediately following the occurrence of the goal-directed behavior. In that case, a written contract, mark on a chart, token system, or some other method can be used to indicate a reward is due. For example, a wall chart could be used to list each activity of daily living (ADL) task to be performed. A mark could be used to indicate 10 minutes of TV time or car riding that could be collected that evening or on the weekend for each task completed.

Some desired behaviors may occur at random or very rarely. In those cases, you can use shaping techniques to reinforce approximations to the target behavior (Berni and Fordyce, 1973). Suppose you hope to teach a new, anxious mother parenting skills. You begin by listing the steps in effective parenting on a chart, and then you demonstrate them to her, e.g., approaching the infant, talking to the infant prior to picking it up, picking the infant up while being careful to provide support for its head, and so on. While doing this demonstration, you ignore the mother's statements of her own fears of failure, thus hopefully extinguishing (or decreasing until it stops) this type of comment. The use of the negative reinforcer of not commenting verbally or nonverbally on the mother's articulated fears will extinguish that behavior in time if you do it consistently. You then ask the mother to copy what you did, praising her for each step she completes successfully. You may also wish to involve the husband, father, or some other significant person. For example, you can get this other person to learn about the chart and praise or otherwise reward the mother too.

Fading is another technique that you can use when teaching new skills. For example, in the case of the anxious mother, as she becomes more confident about picking up and holding the infant, you can decrease your degree of active participation and merely stand by and give her your nonverbal support.

Punishment is relatively ineffective as a technique because it usually has temporary effects, and because it can decrease the rapport that has been established between nurse and client. *Satiation* can help weaken behavior that ordinarily might be punished (Berni and Fordyce, 1973). For example, the natural curiosity of children about matches or curse words can be sated by allowing them to light as many matches at one time in your presence as they want until the urge to do so is dissipated or by asking them to say swear words in front of you until they run out of steam and lose interest. Of course, satiation will only work if you or the family member can allow the behavior to occur in a neutral atmosphere without becoming anxious or punitive. Another alternative to punishment is to reward a behavior that is incompatible with the undesired behavior. For example, rather than punishing a client for overeating, you might reward out-of-the-house activity where food is not available, and thus where the obese client will be less likely to eat.

Extinction is another alternative to punishment. For example, suppose that an elderly client has a habit of cursing that is reinforced by your getting upset and chiding him or her for such behavior. By practicing reacting to the client in a neutral way, you can learn to control your overreaction, and his or her swearing will probably decrease because it is no longer being rewarded by your special attention.

A more effective use of punishment is withdrawal of positive reinforcers. For example, if the child doesn't do his homework, he doesn't get to watch TV, or if the child swears her television privileges are curtailed.

As you work with a client, peer, or yourself, keep visible records of progress from baseline data. These alone will reinforce goal-directed behavior by serving as concrete signs of accomplishment. Written contracts can be used for the same purpose, as well as to underline the seriousness of the client's intent. Figure 8-2 shows an activity behavioral treatment program and contract between client and nurse.

WORKING WITH THE FAMILY

Until recently, parenting was thought to be an innate skill. Now it seems that people do need assistance to learn how to parent. The group setting can be an especially productive learning environment since parents can learn from both you and from one another.

Some skills that you can teach parents (in a group or a three-person session) are how to praise and reward appropriate behavior and how to ignore deviant or inappropriate behavior. Parents can be taught how to use a "time out" period with children where they are taken or sent to their room when inappropriate behavior occurs during a pleasurable event such as watching TV or playing. You can demonstrate how this can be done in a neutral way without threatening, haranguing, or hollering at the child.

Family Resistance to Change

You will probably have to deal with family resistance to methods for instituting behavioral change. One source of resistance to social learning approaches can occur when parental discord and family disorganization are chronic. In these cases, parents provide contradictory cues to their children, and may have difficulty following behavioral prescriptions until the basic parental conflict has been resolved. You may choose to refer these parents to a marital pair psychotherapist who can work with them to resolve the underlying problem.

Another source of resistance can occur when parents insist that all children should be treated alike. Although parents frequently profess this philosophy, they often individualize their children's punishment. One way to deal with this type of resistance is to suggest that social learning methods be practiced with all their children.

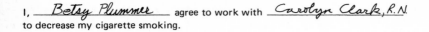

I, _____Betsy Plummer_____ agree to work with _____Carolyn Clark, R.N._____
to decrease my cigarette smoking.

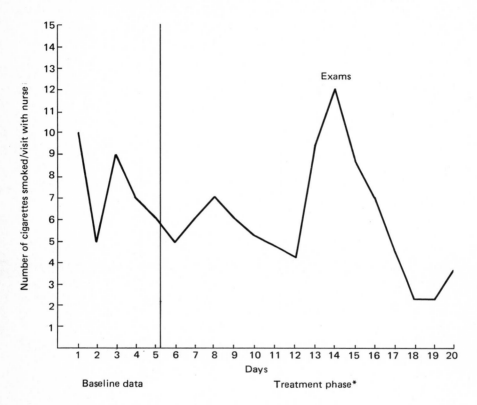

*1 less cigarette than previous visit = nurse will talk with me for 10 extra minutes.

Figure 8-2 An example of a contract and treatment program for one client.

A third source of family resistance is due to the family's need to scapegoat a member. Here, the child's problem behavior serves a highly complex purpose in the family. Thus, if one sibling's behavior is changed through social learning methods, forms of friction or disturbance can occur in other family members. In these instances, you should refer the family to a family therapist who can deal with these more complex interactions.

A nearly universal resistance to social learning methods is the wish not to control another person. Often, it is people who covertly try to control others who protest the most loudly about using systematic, open attempts to control behavior.

Other parents wish to be friends with their children, or hope to be viewed as permissive and accepting. You can present written material to such parents about how parents reward and punish behavior anyway and that shows how social learning methods are merely systematic approaches to changing behavior.

Behavioral Contracts

Families can also be taught how to make contracts for changing behaviors. For example, in a family where the son, Peter, acts up, leaves school, and causes the mother to remain at home more often to check up on him, the following contract might be suggested.

   1 Peter agrees to return to school in exchange for his father working with him on his car.

   2 The mother agrees to spend more time on an individual basis with both Peter and her husband in exchange for being allowed to take a job outside the home.

Families can be taught how to make behavioral contracts like the one above. To do this, you would have to model, shape, explain, prompt, and rehearse clear communication. Harangues, monologues, sermons, and other forms of communication that tend to be tuned out by others need to be shortened and clarified. You would also model and reinforce "I-you" messages such as "I feel . . ." or "I think . . ." and ignore, interrupt, or redirect third-person comments such as, "Oh, he's always like that."

Responsibility for requests and contracts must be limited to the family members who are present at the time the contract is set. Successful contracts require changes "I want" and consequences "I will take responsibility for." In early contract negotiations, you can help the family to discuss alternative rewards or payoffs. For example, in a family where meeting curfew is a problem, alternative ways to meet curfew could include coming home at a prearranged hour, calling a half hour early to negotiate a curfew that is an hour later, averaging curfew times (e.g., out until midnight one night and in by 8 p.m. the next for an average of 10 p.m.), or coming home 1 hour early in exchange for the use of the car (Hardy and Cull, 1974).

Successful contract negotiation requires that ideas such as "I want him to be affectionate" must be translated into specific behaviors such as "husband kisses wife good-bye when leaving for work." It also seems more constructive to focus on contracts that create new behaviors rather than on contracts than emphasize stopping old ones. For example, it is easier to smile than it is to stop frowning, or having one meal together with his family is easier for a certain husband to do than it is for him to stop eating out with the boys altogether (Hardy and Cull, 1974).

Figure 8-3 shows an exercise to use to help clients write and enforce rules for behavior. A more complex skill for you to develop is the ability to train family members to interrupt one another to clarify what was said or to provide each other with feedback on the messages they have received. Because you and the family may seek to hide behind the facade of politeness, this skill may be difficult to acquire. Part of this difficulty seems to be related to a conflict between social role ("I should be polite") and professional role ("I am here to offer a service") and the need of the nurse to be liked or approved of. Working with families, however, requires that you make direct and directive comments in order to produce order and positive growth out of what seems to be chaos and incompatibility (Hardy and Cull, 1974). To begin this process, you may need to make remarks such as: "Ask him to explain that," "Tell her what you think about that," "Before you go on, ask your wife what she feels."

In developing behavioral contracts with families you will need to make assessments with the family, and to assist them to plan small, well-defined changes. Liberman (1970) suggests asking the following questions of all family members as a way to begin specifying behavioral contracts.

1 What changes would you like to see in others in the family?
2 How would you like to be different from the way you are?

You will also need to observe how the family maintains the problematic behaviors. For example, does mother nag father to "control your daughter,"

Figure 8-3 Exercise to Use to Teach Clients How to Write and Enforce Behavioral Contracts in a Constructive Way

Rewrite the following rules in a positive way:

1 If you *don't* do your homework, there'll be *no* TV.
   For example: If you do your homework, you can watch TV.
2 If you *don't* pick your clothes up off the floor, I'll be mad at you.
   For example: If you pick up your clothes 3 days in a row, I'll take you to the movies.
3 If you *don't* stop eating out with the boys, I'll leave you.
   For example: If you eat one meal home with us a week, I'll do your chores.

Write down what the client should do immediately after the desired behavior has occurred.

1 Homework is finished.
   He or she is allowed to watch TV.
2 Clothes are picked up 3 days in a row.
   He or she receives a written or verbal promise to be taken to the movies, followed up by actually being taken to the movies.
3 One meal a week is eaten with family.
   One spouse does the other's chores.

which results in a fight between father and daughter and subsequently in a runaway child who diffuses family tension by leaving the family system? Intervention goals in such a family would probably be to modify behaviors that maintain the delinquent behavior; the father-child arguing could be interrupted by demonstrating and supporting the mother in ways that would help her to reinforce her child's healthy behaviors.

In many cases, deviant behavior in children serves important maintenance functions in the family. These functions must be identified prior to devising an intervention. For example, a teenager who abuses drugs or runs away may serve the purpose of bringing the parents together to focus on their delinquent offspring. Without the teenage behavior, the contact between parents may have remained minimal. A possible behavioral contract in this family is suggested by Hardy and Cull (1974): the teenager is given the freedom to go where he or she wants without questions every day after school in return for a card signed by his or her teacher indicating that school assignments have been completed; the father would monitor the contract (thus meeting the mother's request for more assistance with parenting); and, in return, the father would not be nagged and would receive a bonus of being allowed to go out alone once a week.

Behavioral Rehearsal

Behavioral rehearsal is like a dress rehearsal where you assist clients to practice behaviors that they can use in future situations such as job interviews, shopping trips, social activities, family decisions, or parenting activities (Loomis and Horsley, 1974).

Part of the behavioral rehearsal might be a role-playing situation where you might initially take the role of the client in order to model effective behavior. Or, you may combine role playing with prompting and exploration. The excerpt below shows a role-playing situation where the nurse prompts the client to teach her how to handle social situations where she is anxious about being in a wheelchair.

Nurse: OK. Now pretend we're coming to the picnic and you're in your wheelchair. What happens first?

Client: No one will get out of my way; they won't see me.

Nurse: Tell them, "Excuse me please; may I get through?"

Client: (meekly) Excuse me please, can I come through here?

Nurse: Good. Now say it louder and more firmly.

Client: Excuse me. Let me through please.

Nurse: Very well done. What do you think will happen next?

Client: My leg urinal will be full, but I won't be able to empty it.

Nurse: How could you deal with that?

Client: I don't know.

Nurse: What about asking a person near you to push you to the restroom?

Client: They won't.

Nurse: Try it. You ask me.

Client: Excuse me, could you push me over there?

Nurse: OK. (pause) That worked all right. Now what do you think will happen?

Client: I guess it will work out OK.

SUMMARY

The social learning or behavioral approach focuses on specific, observable behaviors. Since human behavior is learned, it can also be unlearned. There are specific steps that you can take to systematically change behavior and to decrease resistance to this type of approach. Social learning can be used to help individuals to change their habits, to prepare for upcoming situations, and to assist families to be more satisfied with the way their family functions.

PRACTICE EXERCISES

1 Referring to Table 8-1, make a list of behaviors of clients or families you work with that can be counted and that are amenable to a social learning approach.

2 Referring to Figure 8-1, collect baseline data on your own habits in order to modify one of your behaviors.

3 Use Table 8-2 to draw up a list of your own reinforcers.

4 Use Figure 8-2 to draw up a contract indicating your desire to change a behavior, and showing your movement toward that goal; have a colleague or friend sign the contract. Choose someone who will not nag you, but who will support you in your effort to change.

REVIEW

Multiple-Choice Questions

Which of the following behaviors can be counted?

a being affectionate

b taking out the garbage

c not feeling guilty

d completing a report

Matching Terms

Match social learning techniques with the examples by placing the correct letter in front of the appropriate social learning technique.

Social learning techniques	Examples

1 _____ fading

2 _____ expressing countable behaviors

3 _____ rehearsing behavior

4 _____ rewarding appropriate behavior

5 _____ shaping

6 _____ punishing

7 _____ extinguishing a response

a demonstrating and/or rewarding movement toward goal

b practicing for an upcoming situation

c giving a neutral response to a previously rewarded behavior

d smiling

e providing less assistance

f taking away television privileges

g kissing wife good-bye

REFERENCES

Adler, S., and Terry, K. 1972. *Your overactive child: normal or not?* New York: Medcom.

Berni, R., and Fordyce, W. 1973. *Behavior modification and the nursing process.* St. Louis: Mosby.

Carignan, T. 1974. Self-motivation and self-control in operant conditioning. *Perspectives in Psychiatric Care* 12, 1:36–41.

Carruth, B. 1976. Modifying behavior through social learning. *American Journal of Nursing* 76, 11:1804–1806.

Clark, C. 1977. *The nurse as group leader.* New York: Springer.

Durlak, J. 1973. Myths concerning the nonprofessional therapist. *Professional Psychology* 4:300–304.

Gordon, T. 1975. *Parent effectiveness training.* New York: Plume.

Hardy, R., and Cull, J., eds. 1974. *Behavior modification in rehabilitation settings.* Springfield, Ill: Thomas.

Krumboltz, J., and Krumboltz, H. 1972. *Changing children's behavior.* Englewood Cliffs, N.J.: Prentice-Hall.

LeBow, M. 1976. *Approaches to modifying patient behavior.* New York: Appleton-Century-Crofts.

Liberman, R. 1970. Behavioral approaches to family and couple therapy. *American Journal of Orthopsychiatry* 40, 1:106–118.

Loomis, M., and Horsley, J. 1974. *Interpersonal change: a behavioral approach to nursing practice.* New York: McGraw-Hill.

Mash, E. et al., eds. 1976. *Behavior modification approaches to parenting.* New York: Brunner/Mazel.

Robbins, J., and Fisher, D. 1976. *Behavior modification: how to make and break habits.* New York: Dell.

Stuart, R. 1971. Behavioral contracting within families of delinquents. *Journal of Behavior Therapy and Experimental Psychiatry* 2:1–11.

Watzlawick, P. et al. 1974. *Change: Principles of Problem Formation and Problem Resolution.* New York: Norton.

Chapter 9

Community Assessment and Intervention

LEARNING OBJECTIVES

When you finish this chapter, you should be able to:

- List areas to assess in a community
- List essential questions to ask in evaluating resistance to change
- List essential interventions to make to decrease resistance to change

Whether you hope to change the agency within which you work, the client, or a larger system such as a group or community, you need to know how to assess the agency, person, or community and how to use planned change intervention techniques. Although the community will be the example used in developing assessments and interventions, the theory, assessments, and interventions for implementing change should be helpful in your work with both subsystems and larger systems.

ASSESSING THE COMMUNITY

It is wise to remember that the community is not a monolithic structure, but rather is composed of many subsystems that interact and often conflict with one another (Marmor, 1975). To Klein (1968), the community is not a geographical place, but a set of patterned interactions where safety, security, support, and sense of self and significance are derived. In this sense, there are occupational, religious, political, social, and ethnic communities to which a person can belong.

To begin a community assessment you should focus on several areas: who the community is; how needs are met; how deviance and disturbance are handled; how identities are developed; and how community functions are accomplished. You may have already gathered some of this information. Or, you may wish to send out questionnaires, to talk with community representatives or leaders, or to observe how the community looks and operates.

Who and What the Community Is

Your first task is to identify the boundaries of the community. These boundaries may be geographical, social, religious, occupational, educational, health-related, or ethnic. Once boundaries are defined, you may wish to conduct a community survey. This identification is important for several reasons. Crowding conditions and unstable populations can influence the mental and physical health of community members by increasing stress levels. Populations that have specific age, sex, occupational, learning, or family needs that remain unidentified and unmet can also increase stress levels. Communities that cannot provide support and situations where those under stress can test reality decrease the probability of both the physical and mental health of their members. "The key differences between those individuals who experience stress and become sick and those that experience it and do not, involves the opportunity to perform reality testing" (Stress, disease, and the life-support system, *Behavior Today,* 1976). *Reality testing* is the ability to differentiate one's feelings about outer events from the outer events themselves. Clients who have a poor ability to test reality may under- or overreact to external dangers (Brody, 1966; Small, 1971; White, 1974). Significant others who appear calm and concerned provide assistance with reality testing merely by being available and by giving objective information about what is occurring in the external environment. When reality testing is performed in the presence of others, conflict and strain are decreased. A first step in preventing stress is to involve supportive groups such as extended family, peer and religious groups, and clubs and organizations in the reality-testing process. You need to begin to identify the available community support systems for later interventions. Some questions to ask in a community survey are:

- How is space distributed and used? (Where are there highrise buildings, playgrounds and parks, cemeteries, nursing homes, overcrowded areas, natural and physical barriers to social interaction?)
- What are the cultural mix and stability of the population? (Does one set of values and traditions pervade the populations, or are there several cultural groups living in harmony or in conflict, and how much acculturation and stress occur due to people moving in or out of the area?)
- What are the age, sex, and family groupings? (Is this primarily an elderly population, a single-occupancy commuter group, young marrieds with children, or a mix?)
- What income levels are represented and to what extent? (Is this a relatively wealthy population that can afford private health care, a middle-class population that receives little assistance for health care, a poor population that receives governmental or charitable assistance for health care, or is there a mix?)
- What are the occupational levels? (Is the population composed of hard-driving executives who leave the family's health concerns to be managed by their wives? Is this a primarily action-oriented population that learns by doing? Is there a mix? What does occupational level tell you about the population's education, health problems, problem-solving patterns, and methods of learning?)
- What community resources are available and where are they? (Where are the schools, hospitals, shopping areas, and clinics located in relation to available transportation? What self-help or supportive groups and services exist in the community?)

How Needs Are Met

It can be assumed that all human beings have basic needs. Some of these needs may be met or some of them may be prevented from being met by space, culture, age, sex, family, income, occupation level, or community resource factors.

It has been demonstrated that clergy, physicians, and public welfare agencies are more privy to the greatest number of relevant mental health concerns than are mental health agencies or family service centers. It is also known that large numbers of people receive no help at all from professional sources whereas some individuals and families receive an inordinate amount of uncoordinated services from a wide number of agencies. People often have a difficult time asking for help in our society due to strong taboos against being dependent on others (Klein, 1968). All of these factors affect who seeks help to have his or her needs met.

The mental health needs of a population can be identified by asking the community's clergy, physicians, welfare agencies, and clients what needs are not being met.

How Deviance and Disturbance Are Handled

This area covers a wide range of coping devices from the removal of deviants from the community to the social isolation of deviants to the maintenance and support of the person(s) who is deviant within the community. It also entails finding out what the definition of deviance is in the community. Some questions for you to consider in this area are:

- Are people with psychiatric mental health difficulties rejected by the community? In what way?
- How are homosexuals, delinquents, or those who abuse alcohol, drugs, or food treated by community members?
- What political, educational, or social views lead to the rejection of those who deviate from the norm?
- Are there humane or highly institutionalized agencies available in the community to help deal with deviant members? What are they?
- Does the community reject the idea of placing treatment facilities for its deviants within the community? How?
- Is there a prevailing view that people who deviate from accepted behavioral patterns should be punished? How is this belief put into practice?

How Identities Are Developed

Questions in this area deal with identifying the socializing agencies in the community, and studying how they operate, for example:

- How do families teach their members to act?
- What kinds of religious organizations exist in the community and what is their prevailing view of human motivation?
- What youth agencies are there and how do young people relate to them?
- What kind of formal and special education programs are available and how are they used by the community?
- How could already-existing agencies be used more effectively?

How Community Functions Are Accomplished

For community functions to be accomplished, there must be communication, decision making, links between various subsystems, and ways to preserve and strengthen the idea of "community." Some questions to ask to assess this area are:

- Are decisions made before adequate information has been obtained? What possible effect(s) might this have?
- Are decisions made by default, based on the personal concerns of a few, or made by consensus? What are the consequences of this type of decision making?
- Is communication fragmented and inefficient? How does such communication seem to affect the community?
- Are communication messages based on a sense of community (We're all in this together) or on stereotypes and the establishment of distance between groups (It's us against them)? What is the effect of both types of communication message?

- How accurately does the local media portray information to the community?
- Are there informal (rumor) communication channels?
- Are problems solved informally with board and committee meetings used only to record earlier decisions? How might this affect the community or the decision-making process?
- How are ad hoc, neighborhood, or block associations used in decision making?
- How readily are newcomers (including nurses) accepted by the community?
- Is leadership concentrated among a few business and civic groups or is it widely distributed in the community?
- Are there wide vacillations in power or frequent changes in the power base that could affect health planning or treatment?
- Where is power located, how is it perceived, and how is it used?
- What overlapping areas and missing links are there in mental health care services?
- What segments in the community are receptive and hostile to outside influence?
- Is there a sense of trust between community members and leaders?
- Is there community disintegration? [as indicated by a recent disaster affecting the basic means of livelihood for the community, widespread ill health, extensive poverty, confusion of cultural values, weakening of religious affiliations, extensive migration of new groups, and rapid social change affecting traditional patterns of community life (Hughes, 1969)]

RESISTANCE TO CHANGE

Once you have identified the needs of the community and the ways in which it operates you may decide on a course of action. Before acting, you should consider the resistances that you may encounter. Just as a family resists change and attempts to maintain stability or homeostasis, so does the system known as the community.

People who resist change may do so because that change threatens to take away something that they prize. Any threat to the following can lead to people resisting change: current status, existing way of life, job, or money; familiar customs, habits, laws, or rules; and autonomy and free will. Resistance is not always a condition of change. At times it may be a symptom that something is wrong such as the solution is impractical or sufficient rapport has not been established between change agent and clients. To assess sources of resistance, the following questions can be asked:

- What other factors in the system will be affected as a result of the change?
- What forces are operating to inhibit change?
- What information or experiences must precede the change?

- What new procedures or experiences will need to be developed as a result of the change?
- Who is likely to suffer from the change?
- How will power, influence, custom, or life-style be affected by the change?
- How aware is the client of the need for change or of its purpose?
- Is the client sufficiently involved in planning for the change?
- What is the relationship between the change agent and the client?
- What past relationships between the change agent (or agency) and the client might be influencing resistance now?
- How open has the client been to the introduction of change in the past?

If you are planning to introduce change in a community organization, it may help you to know the organizational factors that create the least amount of resistance to change. These factors are free communication, administrative support of and reward for problem-solving efforts, shared decision making, sufficient time to problem-solve, written statements of what the change goals will be, large professional staff, concern with more than just day-to-day operations, staff cohesiveness, physical and social proximity of staff members, history of change, recent change in leadership, no strong vested interests in maintaining the status quo, and feelings of security among individuals (*Planning for Creative Change in Mental Health Services*, 1971).

DECREASING RESISTANCE TO CHANGE

If you can identify the source of resistance, you can intervene at that point. Sometimes it is not possible to locate the source of resistance, or there are many sources of resistance. In such cases you can use the following recommendation for introducing change.

Since the amount of resistance is proportionate to the degree to which people feel threatened, the logical step to take is to reduce the anxiety associated with the change. The measures to reduce anxiety suggested in Chapter 2 can be used. In addition, you can allow people to give vent to their disagreements and conflicts without interrupting them. Nurses seem to view conflict as negative and often try to eliminate it. Conflict and tension can be used in a constructive way if they are assessed and responded to rationally. In order to do this, it will be necessary for you to regard resistance as a natural phenomenon that will gradually decrease with time. As individuals become accustomed to the new ideas they may argue and disagree with one another. This is a useful process as long as you can focus the discussion on the impact of change on the clients (Deloughery, 1971). Conflict will escalate when it is the result of ill-defined goals, lack of information, lack of authority or power to decide, or struggle for status. In such cases, you will need to intervene to provide needed information, to help formulate realistic goals, to establish authority, or to provide rewards for changing.

If you wish to gain support for changes that you introduce, you must be willing to consider modifications in your goals. If you can collaborate and compromise with the client there is a greater chance that at least part of your idea will be implemented and resistance will be reduced (Bennis, 1966). The process of collaborating on goals and working toward them is at least as important as attaining the goals themselves. The more the client can be involved in gathering information about the change and the need for it, the less resistance there will be to the change.

Timing is often an important part of decreasing resistance to change. New ideas should be introduced at a time when the possibility for accepting them seems highest. People are most open to change when there is a crisis, when there is discomfort with the status quo, or when a new leader assumes power.

Besides being aware of the sources of conflict and timing the introduction of change appropriately, you as change agent must be able to inspire confidence that new solutions are possible. The idea that a choice is always available should be promoted. Some comments that can convey this confidence are: "It *is* possible for us to work together to change that" or "I think that if we work together we can plan how to change that." In your communication with clients you should always imply that the responsibility for change rests with them, but that you will assist them to develop methods to change.

Do not assume that resistance to change is always an unrealistic response on the part of your clients. When you confuse your own needs for approval, change, or acknowledgment with the clients' needs, resistance to change is inevitable. Therefore, it is important for you to examine your own needs and to separate them from those of your clients. Although you may be sure that you can provide a needed service for clients, they are always free to accept or reject it.

Resistance to change will be decreased if rewards for changing are given and problem solving is used (see Chapter 8). Support and reward can be developed in group settings. For example, attitude change is more likely to occur when there is an opportunity for people to get to know each other as individuals, when all members are allowed to participate as equals, when there is acceptance of others, and when cooperation rather than competition is encouraged (Wrightsman, 1972). Therefore, when introducing change that will affect a group, it is wise to gather the members of the group together and to structure situations where they can get to know one another and work cooperatively.

The awareness of the need for change occurs much sooner than does the actual change itself. People who change may be perceived as deviant unless the whole system changes at once. However, if opinion leaders in the system accept the change, others may follow (Rogers, 1962). To work with opinion leaders, you must first identify who the leaders in the system are. If possible, it would be beneficial for you to work toward changing the whole system. If this is not possible, you can focus your efforts on opinion leaders and/or on those with high status and work to cause change in them; this change will have a ripple effect and promote change in other parts of the system. Whether you work with the entire client group or with only the opinion leaders, it is necessary that you give them sufficient lead time to understand the change and the need for it and to adjust their thinking to bring it in line with the change.

To influence opinion leaders, you may need to prove your credibility to them as an expert or useful person (Rogers and Shoemaker, 1970). You could do this by explaining how you have assisted others to change, by stating your qualifications, and/or by helping the client to change in some small way and thereby demonstrating your ability to induce change. Perhaps the most significant source of power or influence that you have is your ability to convey concern, to experiment, to be open and honest, to be flexible, to share in decision making, and to cooperate with others; Bennis (1966, p. 169) calls this "value power."

VALUES CLARIFICATION AS PREPARATION FOR CHANGE

One skill that you can teach clients is the ability to guide their own lives based on a valuing process. Possessing such a skill can enable clients to deal with future changes. Clarification of values assists people to work out and make sense of all the information and alternatives that they are exposed to.

In values clarification (Kirschenbaum and Simon, 1974) clients are taught to discover what they prize and cherish. Learning what is valued is both a cognitive and affective process. Discovering what is important to clients necessitates the systematic exploration of what they value. Many people have learned to distrust their own feelings and inner experiences and are not always sure what they *do* prize. Discussing what is prized will clarify this area for both you and the client.

The next step in attaining this skill is to learn how to choose among alternatives. Choosing means learning how to make a realistic examination of the pros and cons of each alternative. Once alternatives are out in the open, clients can make reasonable choices based on the consequences of each alternative. To learn how to choose, clients must be given the chance to make real choices. If you choose and decide for clients, they cannot learn this skill.

Acting on what is valued is a part of the clarification process. People rarely get or take the chance to act on their beliefs and to actualize their full potential. Encouraging planned action enhances the ability of clients to do what they say. When actions are repeated a number of times, patterns are formed, and it is easier to behave in a consistent manner despite contradictory input from the environment. Some questions that you can ask to help clients clarify their values are: "Where did you first get that idea?" "What other alternatives do you have?" "Which alternatives can you reject? Why?" "How do you feel about choosing that solution?" "Who have you discussed (shared) this with?" "How do you plan to implement the action?" "Who will work with you on this?" and "Can I help? How?"

PROVIDING FOR PLANNED CHANGE

Planned change can be divided into phases. The first phase is the development of the need for change. Interventions in this phase include letting clients know that you are available and ready to help them, providing information to sensitize them to specific health concerns, and creating an atmosphere in which the accepted standard is to recognize problems and to deal with them. Comments that you might make are: "I'm ready to work on this problem when you are" "Are you ready to work on _____ problem with me now?" "It seems to me that _____ is a problem that we could work on now" and "Everybody has problems; I'm here to help you work out some of yours."

The second phase is the establishment of a change relationship. Sometimes this phase serves as an evaluation period where you and the client decide whether you can work together. Tasks in this phase include assessing client capacity to accept and use help; assessing your own resources, biases, and potential ability to help; deciding with the client what the expected change entails; anticipating difficulties that may emerge as a result of the change; evaluating your own and the client's coercive or dependent tendencies; and clarifying your own goals in this relationship.

The third phase is the diagnosis of client problems. In this phase, you obtain information by directly questioning and observing your clients. You act cooperatively with the client to encourage analysis of the problem and to teach the client how to identify indicators of problem areas. Some questions that may be useful are: "What do you see as the problem?" and "What makes you aware that there is a problem?"

The fourth phase is the examination of alternate routes and goals for clients. You can help clients to define the direction of change; you can support clients' statements of intent to change, you can provide clients with opportunities for anticipatory testing; and you can teach clients appropriate change behaviors. Some comments that you might make in this phase are: "What alternatives do you have?" "What do you want to change?" "You seem to have decided that you want to change" and "What do you think might happen if you do that?"

The fifth phase is the initiation of the change actions. You role here is to provide support for clients and to develop or stimulate support systems. Helpful comments might be: "You're doing fine" "Who can work with you on this?" and "Who can you talk to for support in this?"

The sixth phase is the stabilization of the change. This includes developing procedures to demonstrate the effects of the change, offsetting resistance to the change, and cultivating the image of the client as someone who has been shown to be capable of change. Some possible comments to this effect are: "You are now more able to deal with _____ as evidenced by _____ " and "You can expect some pressure from

_____ not to change, but that will pass as he or she gets used to your new behavior."

The final phase of planned change is the termination of the client-helper relationship. Prior to ending the relationship, it is suggested that you teach clients how to problem-solve, that you arrange for some other system to take over the functions that you have provided for clients, and that you train clients how and when to seek help (*Planning for Creative Change in Mental Health Services*, 1971).

Throughout any planned change process, you can promote change by assuring that long- and short-term goals and procedures for change are mutually agreed upon, that a review of the progress toward them is conducted periodically, and that the next phase or goal is introduced at the appropriate time. You might say to clients: "You tell me what your idea is about where we are going" and "Let's review what we've achieved. As I see it, we've . . . What is *your* view?"

SUMMARY

In order to assess a community you should focus on who the community is; how needs are met; how deviance and disturbance are handled; how identities are developed; and how community functions are accomplished. Before introducing change into a system, you would be wise to evaluate the sources of resistance to change. Common sources of resistance are fear of loss of current status, existing way of life, job, or money; threat to familiar customs, habits, laws, or rules; and threat to autonomy and free will. Resistance to change can be decreased by decreasing anxiety, by channeling conflict into constructive discussion, by agreeing to modify goals, by using appropriate timing, by inspiring confidence that change can occur, by providing rewards for changing, by working with system leaders, and by proving your credibility as a change agent. You can prepare clients for future changes by teaching them values clarification and by assisting them through a program for planned change.

PRACTICE EXERCISES

1 Conduct a community survey covering all the areas listed under "Assessing the Community."
2 Locate potential sources of resistance in the community or system that you are studying.
3 Make a list of interventions that you can use to decrease resistance to a change that you plan to make.

REVIEW

Listing

1 List areas to assess in a community.

_____

_____

2 List essential questions to ask in evaluating resistance.

_____

_____

_____

_____

_____

_____

_____

3 List essential interventions for decreasing resistance to change.

_____

_____

_____

_____

REFERENCES

Beasley, J. et al. 1973. Community health programming: medical media for the people. _Nursing Digest_ 1, 7:28–32.

Bennis, W. 1966. _Beyond bureaucracy: essays on the development and evolution of human organizations._ New York: McGraw-Hill.

_____ et al., eds. 1969. *The planning of change.* 2d ed. New York: Holt, Rinehart and Winston.

Brody, E. B. 1966. Psychiatry and prejudice. In *American handbook of psychiatry* vol. 3. ed. Silvano Arieti, pp. 629–642. New York: Basic Books.

Budman, S. 1975. A strategy for preventive mental health intervention. *Professional Psychology* 6, 4:394–398.

Deloughery, G. et al., 1971. *Consultation and community organization in community mental health nursing.* Baltimore: Williams and Wilkins.

Fischman, S. 1976. Change strategies and their application to family planning programs. In *Management for nurses, a multidisciplinary approach,* eds. S. Stone et al., St. Louis: Mosby.

Gray, W. et al., eds. 1969. *General systems theory and psychiatry.* Boston: Little, Brown.

House, E. 1976. The micropolitics of innovation: nine propositions. *Phi Delta Kappan* 58, 5:337–340.

Hughes, C. et al. 1969. *People of cove and woodlot: communities from the viewpoint of social psychiatry.* vol. 2. New York: Basic Books.

Kirschenbaum, H., and Simon, S. 1974. Values and the futures movement in education. In *Learning for tomorrow: the role of the future in education,* ed. A. Toffler, New York: Vintage Books.

Klein, D. 1968. *Community dynamics and mental health.* New York: Wiley.

Knight, J. 1974. Applying nursing process in the community. *Nursing Outlook* 22, 11:708–711.

Kohnke, M. et al. 1974. *Independent nurse practitioner.* Garden Grove, Calif.: Trainex.

Marmor, J. 1975. The relationship between systems theory and community psychiatry. *Hospital and Community Psychiatry* 26, 12:807–811.

Planning for creative change in mental health services: a distillation of principles on research utilization. 1971. vol. 1. NIMH. DHEW Pub. #(HSM) 71-9060.

Rodgers, J. 1976. Change process: theoretical considerations involved in the process of change. In *Management for nurses, a multidisciplinary approach,* eds. S. Stone et al., St. Louis: Mosby.

Rogers, E. 1962. *Diffusion of innovation.* New York: Free Press.

_____ and Shoemaker, F. 1970. *Communication of innovations: a cross-cultural approach.* New York: Free Press.

Signell, K. 1975. Training nonprofessionals as community instructors: a mental health education model of primary prevention. *Journal of Community Psychology* 3, 4:365–373.

Small, L. 1971. *The Briefer Psychotherapies.* New York: Brunner/Mazel.

Spradley, B., ed. 1975. *Contemporary community nursing.* Boston: Little, Brown.

Stress, disease, and the life-support system. 1976. *Behavior Today* 7, 42:3.

Watzlawick, P. et al. 1974. *Change: principles of problem formation and problem resolution.* New York: Norton.

Weiss, S., ed. 1975. *Proceedings of the national heart and lung institute working conference on health behavior.* DHEW Pub. #(NIH) 76-868.

White, R. W. 1974. Strategies of adaptation: an attempt at systematic description. In *Coping and adaptation*, ed. George V. Coelho, David A. Hamburg, and John E. Adams, pp. 47–68. New York: Basic Books.

Wrightsman, L. 1972. *Social psychology in the seventies*. Monterey, Calif: Brooks/Cole.

Part Two

Observation and Communication Guides

Chapter 10

Process Recordings

LEARNING OBJECTIVES

When you finish this chapter, you should be able to:

- Define process recording
- Identify nonfacilitative nurse comments
- Identify facilitative nurse comments

A *process recording* is a verbatim, sequential report of the client's verbal and nonverbal communication, of the nurse's verbal and nonverbal communication, and of the nurse's analysis, evaluation, and speculations about the communications.

USES OF PROCESS RECORDINGS

Although writing down what occurs in a nurse-client interaction is often tedious and time-consuming, process recordings can be invaluable. They provide a permanent record of what took place. Since recall diminishes rapidly with time, a written record can prove helpful in jogging your memory. Also, since most of us have a tendency to censor and/or to forget anxiety-provoking interactions, a written record can serve to preserve a more complete sense of what took place.

Process recordings show the process or flow of what took place. Thus, it is possible to examine how you responded each time the client showed anxiety or anger, and how communication patterns between you and the client were reinforced.

Process recordings allow you to study your communication skills within an interview and over time. For example, if you complete a process recording for the first, middle, and last interview with a client, you can compare how your ability to communicate with the client has decreased or increased from interview to interview. Often, this kind of analysis can give you clues to what blocks communication, to what kinds of comments seem to lead to increased or decreased distance between you and the client, and to what kinds of idiosyncratic speech patterns you have.

This type of recording can also be used to present clinical data for a group conference or individual supervisory session. In the former case, you may wish to extract portions of a word-for-word conversation as a way to illustrate to your peers the assessments, interventions, or difficulties that you have developed with a specific client. In the latter case, a psychiatric mental health nursing consultant or specialist may request specific blow-by-blow interchanges; consultation or clinical supervision requires specific communication as it occurred because although there are certain communication principles, their specific application is determined by each unique relationship. Thus, in order for another to suggest alternate interventions, it is necessary to have the specific verbal and nonverbal communication of both you and the client in the context within which it occurred.

SAMPLE PROCESS RECORDINGS

Figure 10-1 shows a process recording a community health nurse completed while interviewing a 28-year-old white male client who had recently been discharged from the hospital after having had a total hip replacement. Because this recording was to be presented to the mental health consultant, the community health nurse did not add written reactions or self-analysis of her own comments. It is possible, and often preferable, to add a column entitled, "Self-analysis" or "Self-evaluation" where you can place your own (subjective) reactions to what you and the client said or did. For further instructions in this method see Clark (1975; 1977). The client had had severe rheumatoid spondylitis for several years. The first time the nurse visited him, she noticed that the client did not seem motivated to complete postsurgical exercises or to resume activities of daily living. In fact, the client was characterized by the nurse as "depressed"

Figure 10-1 Process Recording with a 28-Year-Old White Male Who Had Just Had a Total Hip Replacement

Nurse-client interchange	Consultant's comments
Nurse: Hi. How are you?	
Client: Oh, not too bad.	
Nurse: What have you been doing?	
Client: Oh, nothing; I just got through eating.	*Is nurse anxious? a switch here to safe topic, the weather.*
Nurse: Isn't the weather nice? Are you planning to go outside today?	
Client: Yes, if it doesn't rain.	
Nurse: What do you mean?	*good; a facilitative comment.*
Client: It seems whenever I want to go out it starts to rain.	*Theme?: things go wrong for me.*
Nurse: Oh, do you think it's bad luck?	*Might ask for "an example of one time things went wrong."*
Client: I don't know—maybe. Let's hope it doesn't rain all summer.	*Unclear question and a change of topic.*
Nurse: Let's see, it's going to be a year this summer, isn't that right?	
Client: Yes.	
Nurse: Are you still on disability?	*Yes-no question.*
Client: No.	
Nurse: How are you managing?	*Did the client miss the point of your question? If so, restate, e.g. "How are things going?"*
Client: On welfare.	
Nurse: Oh, is that enough for your expenses?	
Client: Yeah, it's enough.	
Nurse: Do you pay rent on your apartment?	*Yes-no questions. Might try, "How do you get your meals?"*
Client: Yes, but it's not very much and I don't need things anymore.	
Nurse: How about food? Do you give anything toward that?	
Client: No. She has to cook meals all different times of the day and there usually is something I can eat. She has to cook for the kids and then when my sister comes home from work she cooks again.	*Client begins to talk more freely at this point. Could it be the topic and/or his level of anxiety?*
Nurse: My, your mother is a hard worker, just like your father.	*Judgmental comment: He doesn't quite agree as he says, she works "pretty hard"; this shows he is able to disagree.*
Client: Yeah, she works pretty hard.	
Nurse: How have you been feeling?	
Client: Oh, my neck is still stiff, but the doctor said it would take a while for the medicine to take effect. My bad leg is fine but I'm worried about my left leg.	
Nurse: Why?	*Good. You're exploring.*
Client: I still have some pain in the upper part of my leg where the spasm was and the doctor said part of the pain is caused by arthritis. I'm worried because it comes and goes. Maybe I'll have to have the other one operated on. The trouble is, there's no way of knowing. But, I still worry.	

Figure 10-1 Process Recording with a 28-Year-Old White Male Who Had Just Had a Total Hip Replacement (*Continued*)

Nurse-client interchange	Consultant's comments
Nurse: So, have you been doing anything new besides walking around, sitting, and watching the children?	*Are only "new" things important? Be careful of putting your own values in.*
Client: NO-o-o-o-o.	
Nurse: What about these books and magazines that are here on the floor?	
Client: Oh, I've been looking at them, and reading some dopey stories like the ones in *Modern Screen* and *True Story*.	
Nurse: Some of the stories in those magazines are really dopey. Don't you think so?	*I wonder why you said this since he had just said he thought this was true. What about, "What's dopey about them?"*
Client: Yeah-h-h-h-h. I finally finished a book I've been reading.	
Nurse: What was it about?	
Client: It's about a colored girl who was almost white and how she goes down south to look for her boyfriend and the trouble she gets into and how she gets thrown into jail for no reason at all. I wouldn't recommend it.	
Nurse: Why not?	
Client: Well, the author went on and on describing things like scenery and I ended up skimming a lot of it.	
Nurse: Well, it's good to see you're slowly beginning to improve. Are you able to help yourself more?"	*Might be more helpful to describe exactly what he is doing to improve and/or ask, "How do you see your progress?"*
Client: No. Getting up is still hard, but I can get into bed by myself.	
Nurse: Do you watch much TV?	
Client: Only for 2 or 3 hours at night. I like to watch Johnny Carson, but I have to go to bed when my father gets home.	*Might ask, "How come?" Couldn't he arrange to stay up later with your help?*
Nurse: Well, then, it will be good when you can help yourself more.	
Client: Yeah, but I guess I'm not so bad off when you see some others who are worse off than me. My roommate was paralyzed from the waist down. He keeps thinking he can walk again.	*This sounds like a rationalization.*
Nurse: Well, it does make you wonder why things like that happen.	*You seem to be conveying that you think he or others got a bad deal. Do you feel helpless or hopeless re this client?*
Client: Yeah, I guess so but I guess it's just something you have to take. But some people never get sick . . .	

and "frustrating to work with." The psychiatric mental health nursing consultant suggested that the nurse complete a process recording during her next visit to the client. The result of the visit appears in Figure 10-1. The consultant's comments and suggestions appear opposite the transcription of the community health nurse's recording.

In general, the nurse-client interaction progresses from a beginning point where the nurse makes social conversation and asks questions that can be answered with a yes or a no, to a midpoint where more facilitative questions such as "How have you been feeling?" "What was it about?" and "Why was that?" encourage the client to expand his comments. By looking at this brief interview, it is possible to see how the nurse can influence the client's comments merely by asking a type of question that facilitates client communication.

In Figure 10-2 another nurse-client interchange is recorded. This time, the interaction was recorded because the nurse verbalized a wish to improve her skills of talking with a married couple. Because three people are involved, it is possible to identify some elements of the family system. For example, Mrs. W attempts to triangle in the nurse. This interview also progresses from a beginning point where the nurse deals with her own anxiety by making social comments, changing topics, and apologizing. As nurse and clients become less anxious, all

Table 10-1 Facilitative and Nonfacilitative Nurse Comments

Nonfacilitative comments	Facilitative comments
"Are you tired?"	"What are you feeling?"
"You haven't been working, right?"	"Tell me about your work history."
"Do you get along with your parents?"	"Tell me a little about you and your parents."
"It's good that you try to get along with them."	"How do you see the progress you've made?"
"Do you watch much television?"	"What television programs do you watch?"
"I can't understand why she'd say that to you!"	"What do you make of your mother saying that?"
"I want you to do . . ."	"What health goals can we work on together?"
"I'm sorry if I caused a problem."	"You seem to have some feelings about that; let's talk them over."
"Let's talk about something else."	"What would you like to talk about?"
"You're right; death is a morbid subject."	"Talking about death may be difficult, but in the long run it can help you to deal with it."

Figure 10-2 Process Recording with Mr. and Mrs. W. Mrs. W is 69 Years Old and Has Metastatic Cancer. Mr. W Is 79 Years Old and Has Cardiac Involvement.

Nurse-client interchange	Consultant's comments
Nurse (Mrs. L): (standing at doorway) How about the sale of your apartment? Have you heard anything?	
Mr. W: We haven't done anything about it.	
Mrs. W: What do you mean "we"? I have, you haven't.	
Mr. W: (walks out of apartment)	You might encourage him to stay, e.g., "Let's discuss this."
Mrs. W: He can't make a decision about anything. Always the nice guy. I do the dirty work and everyone likes him. He doesn't like to talk. There's nothing I can do. I just give up!	"You have some feelings about this?"
Nurse: I'm sorry if I caused a problem.	Are you meeting your own need to be approved of? I suspect this problem is unrelated to you.
Nurse: I would like to know how he feels though. Maybe the three of us could talk things over.	Good comment. Although they do not respond here, they take you up on your offer later.
Mrs. W: He has a terrible temper when he gets upset and at those times you just leave him alone. This leaves me up in the air.	Is she telling you to be careful and not introduce change? This seems like a subtle threat that if you try to talk, something terrible will happen.
Nurse: What did the lawyer say?	
Mrs. W: He said Mr. W's concern was for me and that he shouldn't concern himself with his daughter. Maybe when he sees that he needs this money to take care of me he will do something.	Theme: I want him to be more concerned about me.
Mr. W: (returns; begins to open and close drawers in the kitchen)	You might say "Come and join us Mr. W."
Nurse: Let's get that financial report and see if I can help you with that.	
Mrs. W: (gets report) This is really hard to figure.	
Mr. W: (passing through room on way to bathroom) You don't have to have it to the penny.	Mr. W seems to want to get involved in the discussion.
Mrs. W: (looking at report, whispering) I don't how much of this will change because of the cancer.	
Nurse: Why are you whispering?	Good; brings nonverbal message into the open for discussion.
Mrs. W: I don't want to upset him. He was so upset when he first found out.	"What was your reaction to his upset?"
Nurse: (goes over to bathroom door) What are you fixing, Mr. W?	Good; Trying to get him involved. Otherwise he might think you're trying to side with his wife.
Mrs. W: That's the holder I broke when I fell.	

Figure 10-2 Process Recording with Mr. and Mrs. W. Mrs. W is 69 Years Old and Has Metastatic Cancer. Mr. W Is 79 Years Old and Has Cardiac Involvement. (*Continued*)

Nurse-client interchange	Consultant's comments
Nurse: Things keep you busy around here.	*Unrelated comment. It might be more useful to say, "What happened when you fell?"*
Mr. W: Yes, there's always plenty to do.	
Mrs. W: Mrs. L, would you like to talk to the two of us?	
Mr. W: What do you want to talk about?	
Nurse: Well, Mrs. W and I have been doing a lot of talking about the present and also about your plans for the future. I'm interested in how you think and feel.	*Good.*
Mr. W: There certainly is a lot to think about the future. The future will have to be worked out.	*"Perhaps we can plan for it."*
Nurse: How about now?	
Mr. W: Well, we're doing all right. I think right now things are OK. You certainly have been a help.	*"What do you think about what your husband said?" (to Mrs. W.)*
Nurse: What about your plans to go to Florida?	
Mr. W: Well, I'd like to go. I know some people who can stay here. I won't leave you completely stranded.	
Mrs. W: I thought you wanted someone here all the time! And what about someone going with you?	*"What is your reaction to your husband wanting to go to Florida?"*
Mr. W: That's no problem. My nephew can go down with me. He can come back by plane.	
Nurse: I saw some ads in the paper Sunday about household help.	*Good. Goal-directed activity. Be careful of imposing your values. Might be better to help the two of them plan together with your guidance.*
Mr. W: (gets paper to look for ads)	
Nurse: (to Mrs. W when Mr. W has left) Maybe you should let him plan things.	*"Has that happened?" "What were the circumstances?"*
Mrs. W: I can't. He won't do anything.	

are able to focus more constructively on the tasks of communicating and decision making. Table 10-1 lists some nurse statements that are likely to facilitate communication and some that are likely to block communication. For an indepth discussion of communication skills and interviewing techniques, see Clark (1977, pp. 229–290).

SUMMARY

Process recordings are verbatim, sequential reports of the client's verbal and nonverbal communication, of the nurse's verbal and nonverbal communication, and of the nurse's analysis, evaluation, and speculations about the communications. Although tedious to complete, process recordings can provide the nurse with helpful information about how to improve nurse-client communication.

PRACTICE EXERCISES

1 Choose two clients with whom you are having difficulty relating.
2 Do a 5-minute process recording with each.
3 Examine each recording for facilitative and nonfacilitative comments.
4 Show the recordings to a peer, supervisor, or consultant for the purpose of eliciting more communication suggestions.
5 Do two more 5-minute process recordings with the clients; this time try to implement what you learned.

REVIEW

Define process recording.

_____

_____

_____

Matching Terms

Match nonfacilitative nurse comments with their restatements by placing the correct letter in front of the appropriate nonfacilitative comment.

Nonfacilitative comments	Facilitative comments
1 _____ "Are you angry?"	a "What do you think she meant by that remark?"
2 _____ "That's good."	b "What would you like to discuss?"
3 _____ "Do you like your husband?"	c "What do you think about your progress?"
4 _____ "What a silly thing for her to say to you!"	d "What are you feeling now?"
5 _____ "Let's not talk about that."	e "How are things between you and your husband?"

REFERENCES

Clark, C. C. 1975. *Recording and evaluating nurse-patient interactions: using the process recording guide.* Garden Grove, Calif.: Trainex.
_____ 1977. *Nursing concepts and processes.* Albany: Delmar.

Chapter 11

Mental Health
Assessment/Intervention

LEARNING OBJECTIVES

When you finish this chapter, you should be able to:

- List common mental health problem areas
- List areas to assess when making a mental health assessment

Mental health assessments can be made in a number of ways. Only one method will be presented here. This method is based on a problem-oriented approach. The problems listed are ones that seemed to occur most frequently in two community health nursing agencies (see Table 11-1). In the Problem-Oriented Record (POR) system, a problem is any specific difficulty that interferes with the client's highest level of wellness. The POR is meant to assure that none of the client's problems are glossed over. In psychiatric mental health PORs, strengths and healthy aspects of the individual are also listed, as are untapped resources within self, family, or community (Mazur, 1974).

Table 11-1 Mental Health Assessments and Interventions

Assessment area (Problem)	Goals	Interventions
Orientation	Establish working relationship	Set limits of relationship Reinforce limits Follow through on agreed-upon goals
Anxiety	Decrease anxiety	Prepare client for upcoming events Teach client relaxation exercise(s) Teach client to identify source(s) of anxiety Teach client to recognize body clues associated with high anxiety Remain present Decrease client's sensory stimulation Use concise, infrequent comments that orient and direct client Point out reality to client Encourage client to express feelings
Suicidal potential	Promote life	Explore client's suicidal thoughts, feelings, and/or plans Help establish supportive interpersonal network for suicidal client
Coping devices	Strengthen coping responses	Point out client's strengths Point out client's progress toward goal Teach client adaptive behaviors Prepare client for upcoming events Implement behavior modification program Promote separateness of family members Teach client parenting skills Teach client to develop behavioral contracts with others Role play interpersonal situations Teach client to summarize progress toward goal
Conflict	Resolve conflict	Teach client to examine parts of conflict Support constructive aspects of conflict behavior Assist client to make effective decisions
Communication	Improve communication skills	Clarify unclear statements Use silence Model effective communication Use structured communication exercises Reinforce effective communication Validate messages with client

Table 11-1 Mental Health Assessments and Interventions (*Continued*)

Assessment area (Problem)	Goals	Interventions
Grief/loss/ depression	Assist with grief process	Encourage client to express thoughts and feelings Implement behavioral modification program Include family/friends in plans and interventions
Dependency/ problem solving	Promote problem solving	Ask client to describe a particular interpersonal event in detail Give information as necessary Ask client to state ideas Teach client decision-making skills Set up situations where client can practice new behavior patterns
Family interaction	Promote family interaction	Teach family members to share thoughts, feelings, ideas, and/or activities with each other
	Promote family separateness	Introduce and/or support interactions with extra family members
Termination of nurse-client relationship	Teach client to separate from others effectively	Begin to prepare client for end of nurse-client relationship at beginning of relationship Spend time summarizing and evaluating nurse-client relationship with client Encourage client to explore past separations and their relationship to this one

PROBLEM-ORIENTED MENTAL HEALTH NURSING RECORDS

The first step in a problem-oriented mental health nursing record is the initial assessment. This assessment provides a data base from which to work (Bonkowsky, 1972). Table 11-2 shows an initial assessment for one client.

Once a data base has been collected, a problem list can be developed. Table 11-3 shows a problem list that was developed based on the initial assessment.

The problem list can be attached to the inside cover of the client's record. This allows the reader to have a quick overview of the types of nursing interventions that may be needed.

A Course of Nursing Treatment sheet can be used to chart the focus of nursing visits during the nurse-client relationship. Figure 11-1 shows this course for the client used to illustrate the initial assessment and problem list.

Table 11-2 Initial Mental Health Assessment

	Name _Samuel Fun_	
	Age _68_	
	Date of assessment _2/19/77_	

Assessment area	Questions to ask/ assessments to make	Client's responses	Impression of problem/strengths
Client's view of treatment	"How do you think I can be of help to you?" or "What are you expecting us to work on?"	"I don't know how you can help beside taking my B/P."	The client may need orientation to services that a community health nurse can offer.
Client's goals for treatment	"What do you want to achieve?" or "How can I help you to feel better (be healthier, do more)?"	"I want to be able to get out of the house more."	This is a strength; the client is able to state an observable goal.
Client's self-view	"Describe yourself to me" or "If you had to tell me about yourself in one or two sentences, what would you say?"	"I'm one of the best." "I can't talk with people easily."	The client may have mixed feelings about himself, and he may be questioning his ability to relate to me. Wondering if he can talk with me is an expected reaction at the beginning of a nurse-client relationship.
Recent changes or losses	"What in your life has changed in the past year?" or "What have you lost or gained this year?"	"My best friend, Rob, died last year."	There is possible unresolved grief present.
Physical complaints	"What eating difficulties (patterns) do you have?" and "What sleeping difficulties (patterns) do you have?" and "What elimination problems do you have?" and "What other physical problems (complaints) do you have?"	"I eat OK, but I lost 30 lbs. since Christmas." "I sleep, but I wake up real early." "I'm constipated."	There is possible depression present.

Table 11-2 Initial Mental Health Assessment (*Continued*)

Assessment area	Questions to ask/ assessments to make	Client's responses	Impression of problem/strengths
Other therapies	"What drugs do you take?" and "What other treatments or therapies are you using?"	"I don't take no drugs." No response.	
Feeling difficulties	"What do you do when you get tense or upset to calm down?" and "How do you know when you're upset or angry?" and/or "What do you feel inside when you're upset?" or "People feel tension in different parts of their body; where do you feel tension?"	"I never get nervous." "The last time I was angry was when I played baseball as a kid." No response. No response. "I don't watch television because it's violence, violence!" (spontaneous comment)	The client is denying his feelings. The client is sensitive to expressions of feeling in the external environment. He may be repressing his anger.
Thought difficulties	By this point in the interview, it should be clear whether the client understands the questions asked, whether his comments seem logical and related to yours, and whether he is having difficulty organizing his thoughts. If not, you can ask: "Which of my questions are hard for you to answer?" "Why?" "How has your memory been lately?" In addition if the client seems depressed, has a high suicide potential (see Chapter 4), or mentions wanting to die, you can ask him: "Have you been thinking of killing yourself?" or "What thoughts about suicide have you had?"	"I never think about dying; it's too morbid."	The client seems to misunderstand and/ or not to hear or be able to answer some of my questions. Denial and/or cerebral vascular changes could be influencing his ability to concentrate and communicate clearly.

Table 11-2 Initial Mental Health Assessment (*Continued*)

Assessment area	Questions to ask/ assessments to make	Client's responses	Impression of problem/strengths
Action difficulties	"What difficulties do you have in doing what you want to do?" and "What problems in moving do you have?"	"I'm slower than I used to be." The client was returning to his unmade bed as I left. He walks slowly and shows signs of fatigue or effort in moving.	The client may be showing signs of psychomotor retardation; aging; hopelessness; withdrawal/isolation; weakness due to weight loss.
Communication difficulties	"What problem do you have in talking to people?" and "What problems are you having in talking to me?"	"Nothin' to say." "I can't hear or see too good." "Nobody's here during the day." No response.	The client may have difficulty receiving and sending messages due to sensory deprivation, decreased interpersonal stimulation, and insufficient learning regarding how to communicate his thoughts and feelings.
Relationships with others	"Who are you closest to?" or "Who is your best friend?" or "Who can you confide in?"	"I'm not close to anyone." "I used to be able to talk to Rob." No eye contact with me; flat affect when speaking	The client has few or no sources of interpersonal support; is he still grieving?
Developmental difficulties	Use Erikson's developmental tasks* to assess this area by listening to and observing the client. It may take more than one visit to complete your assessment.		Is the client having feelings of despair, mistrust, and/or isolation?

157

Table 11-2 Initial Mental Health Assessment (*Continued*)

Assessment area	Questions to ask/ assessments to make	Client's responses	Impressions of problems/strengths
Coping devices and strengths	Listen to client and use referral information to make this assessment.		The client uses denial to deal with feelings; he takes to bed (withdrawal) when anxious or hopeless. He lives with Tom and Kate D. who expressed their concern for the client and/or the need for help by calling the agency and requesting a home visit from a nurse.
Goals for the future	"What are you looking forward to?" or "What are your goals for the future?" or "What are you hoping to accomplish?"	No response. "I don't have any." "Nothing."	The client may be depressed; he may also be showing signs of learned helplessness.

*Erik H. Erikson. 1963. *Childhood and Society.* 2d ed. New York: Norton.

It is suggested that the nurse write down assessment areas (and potential questions to ask or assessments to make if necessary) on a piece of paper or 5″ × 8″ card for use during the interview. Some clients will volunteer much or all of the assessment information, others will present it in different order and/or may need to be asked about some of the areas, and others will need to be asked questions in order for them to focus on mental health considerations.

Table 11-3 Problem List

		Client *Samuel Fan*	
Current and active problems	**Noted**	**Date**	**Resolved**
1 Grief	2/19/77		
2 Orientation	2/19/77		4/15/77
3 Anxiety	2/19/77		
4 Conflict	4/3/77		
5 Communication	2/19/77		

For some visits, you may not wish to write narrative notes. This may occur when you focus on the same problem in several visits. The sample Course of Nursing Treatment for Iris Winters shows that a narrative record was kept on 12/3, 12/9, 12/16, 12/28, 1/3, and 1/20. Figure 11-2 shows the narrative record for one visit.

Some community health agencies use a Nursing Care Plan sheet. A portion of the nursing care plan for Iris Winters is shown in Figure 11-3.

SUMMARY

A problem-oriented mental health nursing record is based on an initial assessment. In order to make this assessment, you can use a problem list in collaboration with a course of treatment sheet, a nursing care plan, and narrative records.

Figure 11-1 Course of Nursing Treatment

Name _Iris Winter_

Number and date of visit

Problem/Intervention	1	2	3	4	5	6	7	8	9	10	11	12	13	14	15	16	17	18	19
	12/3/76	12/5	12/7	12/9	12/14	12/16	12/19	12/20	12/22	12/24	12/28	12/30	1/2/77	1/3	1/5	1/7	1/9	1/14	1/20
	n*			n*		n*					n*								n*
Orientation	√	√	√																
Anxiety	√	√	√	√	√	√	√		√				√						
Coping devices		√	√√	√		√	√	√√	√										
Communication							√√	√√			√√	√	√	√					
Dependency/Problem Solving							√√				√√√					√√		√	√
Terminate nurse-client relationship	√													√		√√		√	√

Nurse's signature

Carolyn Clark, R.N.
C.C., R.N.
C.C., R.N.
C.C., R.N.
C.C., R.N.
C.C., R.N.
C.C., R.N.
C.C., R.N.
C.C., R.N.
C.C., R.N.
C.C., R.N.
C.C., R.N.
C.C., R.N.
C.C., R.N.
C.C., R.N.
C.C., R.N.
C.C., R.N.
C.C., R.N.
C.C., R.N.

*n = narrative

160

Figure 11-2 Nurse's Notes

Name _Iris Winter_ Doctor _Pond_

Date and time

12/19

1 p.m.

For first time, client initiated spontaneous discussions of experiences which evoke anxiety for her. She seems quite worried about displeasing her daughter, and seems to be converting this anxiety into tension headaches. Plan to work with client in a problem-solving effort focused on ways to decrease her anxiety.

Carolyn Clark, R.N.

Figure 11-3   Nursing Care Plan

Name ___Iris Winter___

Date	Problem	Goal	Intervention	Evaluation of intervention
12/3/76	Anxiety	to decrease anxiety	relaxation exercises	12/9/76 Anxiety decreased (increased eye contact and discussion of feelings; "I feel better.")
			exploration of interpersonal situations that evoke anxiety	
12/3/76	Orientation	to establish nurse-client relationship	gave information about purpose	12/5/76 client seems motivated to work with me ("I think you can help me.")
12/5/76	Communication	to help client learn to describe thoughts and feelings	exploration of thoughts and feelings	12/5/76 client made some progress (was able to describe an interaction with her daughter where she felt highly anxious. Will continue to work with client on this problem.)

PRACTICE EXERCISES

1 Use Table 11-2 to do a mental health assessment of several clients.
2 Develop problem lists and nursing care plans for the clients.

REVIEW

Listing

1 List common mental health problem areas.

_____

_____

_____

2 List areas to assess when making a mental health assessment.

_____

_____

_____

_____

_____

REFERENCES

Bonkowsky, M. 1972. Adapting the POMR to community child health care. *Nursing Outlook* 20, 8:515–518.

Gerken, Betty; Molitor, Annette M.; and Reardon, James D. 1974. Problem-oriented records in psychiatry. *NCNA* 9, 2:289–302.

Kelly, Mary E., and McNutt, Harland. 1974. Implementation of problem-oriented charting in a public health agency. *NCNA* 9, 2:281–287.

Mazur, Wladyslaw Piotr. 1974. *The problem-oriented system in the psychiatric hospital: a complete manual for mental health professionals.* Garden Grove, Calif.: Trainex.

Yarnall, Stephen R., and Atwood, Judith. 1974. Problem-oriented practice for nurses and physicians. *NCNA* 9, 2:215–228.

Chapter 12

Family Observation and Assessment Guide

LEARNING OBJECTIVES

When you finish this chapter, you should be able to:

- List eleven areas of family assessment
- Identify examples of assessments to be made in each area

As a community health nurse, you have a unique opportunity to observe families in their own environment. Families will often show you aspects of themselves the nurse who works in a hospital or clinic may never see. Because of this unique perspective, you are the logical practitioner to work with families to encourage healthy communication patterns, to prevent mental health difficulties, and to teach family members effective ways to relate with one another.

Being allowed to enter family systems in this way is both an asset and a liability. Try to make sure that you do not become part of the family system; such an involvement on your part will lead to your feeling anxious, conflicted, frustrated, and, possibly, guilty. One way to reduce the potential for getting caught up in family dynamics is to make initial assessments of families in order to identify potential ways in which families may try to involve you in their interaction.

Family assessments are made in the same way that individual assessments are made of the identified patient. The identified patient is the person who is referred to the community health agency; frequently other family members have as many if not more health needs.

You will probably work with families to teach family members how to care for the identified patient, to help family members make rational decisions about health care, and to be a model for effective communication. Because of your work in these areas, knowing how to assess family interaction can be an asset than can enhance your teaching skills.

WHAT TO OBSERVE IN THE FAMILY VISIT

There are at least eleven areas of family functioning that can be observed and assessed. They range from very basic considerations like who is present during the visit to seating arrangement, anxiety levels, family norms, critical events, family roles, functional and dysfunctional family relationships, leadership, disruptions, general atmosphere, and phases of interaction. These areas will be discussed individually, and then the "Family Observation and Assessment Guide will be presented"; this guide will enable you to gather together information from all areas of assessment.

Who is Present

The first thing to observe is who is present when you enter the home. This observation may be made automatically. In other cases, it may force you to become aware that certain family members are always or never present when you visit the identified patient.

Of course, some family members may be at work or in school when you visit. Others may be in the house, but may stay out of your sight. Some of them may be listening to what is said, while others may not seem to be interested in your visit.

Other family members may seem to always want to be present when you visit. They may try to make sure that you and the identified patient are never left alone. Such behavior can have several meanings. For example, the family member might be trying to provide support for the patient. Or, the family member may be seeking support or attention from you. Another meaning is that the family member does not think that the identified patient is capable of speaking up for herself. Still another meaning is that the family member wants to control what the identified patient says to you, and make sure that she does not share family secrets with you.

Seating Arrangement

Drawing a diagram of how you and the family sit or stand can be helpful in a number of ways. First, if it is done for a number of visits, a pattern may begin to emerge. For example, you may find that you always sit between the identified patient and his wife. This seating arrangement may perpetuate a pattern where the identified patient speaks to you and the wife speaks to you, but they never speak to one another. In many cases, you may wish to encourage communication between them and to decrease the potential for putting yourself in the middle.

When one community health nurse did a "Family Observation and Assessment Guide," she began to realize that part of her feeling of being pressured to side with the husband against the wife was a result of the way they sat during the visits. After consultation with the mental health nursing specialist, the nurse moved her chair to allow husband and wife to face one another; she also used phrases such as, "Tell your husband what you think" to encourage more direct communication between them. Figure 12-1 shows the seating arrangement before and after the nurse intervened to change a communication pattern that she thought had been ineffective. The arrows show the direction of communication.

By paying attention to where family members sit or stand, you can also discover clues about what possible nursing interventions you should make. For example, in one family, the community health nurse noticed that the mother of the identified patient was never in the same room with the nurse and patient, but shouted directions or comments to them from the kitchen. By diagramming this pattern, the nurse became interested in exploring the meaning and potential ineffectiveness of such a communication pattern. Later, the nurse and patient asked the patient's mother to join them so that what was said could be heard clearly and responded to more completely. This intervention also reduced the nurse's discomfort since she had felt pulled in two directions by trying to bathe the patient and to still listen to the mother's comments from the kitchen.

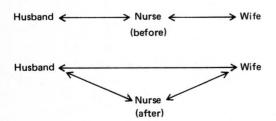

Figure 12-1 Seating arrangement and communication.

Anxiety Levels

By beginning to chart the change in the general level of anxiety during one or more visits, you can begin to see a pattern emerging. Usually, anxiety levels are highest at the beginning of a visit and at the end of a visit. During the middle of many visits, both you and family members may become more comfortable with each other, and have a better idea of what to expect; knowing what to expect often decreases anxiety. As the end of the visit approaches, both nurse and family members may become more anxious; the nurse because she has to find a gracious way to end the visit and leave, and the patient or family member because he or she has more to say or wishes to receive more support from you, or wishes the visit to end but feels guilty about having such a wish. As you visit families, you may want to observe whether your visits follow this common pattern, or whether a different one emerges. (If necessary, refer to Chapter 2, "Anxiety," for a review of the process of assessing anxiety.)

Family Norms

Norms are rules for behavior. Family members develop ways to relate to one another, and certain subjects or behaviors are labeled as acceptable or unacceptable for that family. Such topics of conversation or behaviors are often assumed by family members to be unacceptable for nonfamily members, such as the nurse.

When you enter a home and refuse coffee that is offered to you in a family where the norm is to share coffee, you may be violating an important family norm. Going along with a family norm like sharing coffee may be important and useful, whereas going along with a family norm like not talking about death and dying in a family where a member is dying may not be useful. Before you can know what the family's norms are, you have to watch and listen for clues. Each family has ways in which it enforces its rules and maintains or reestablishes homeostasis. For example, the mother may scowl at the son if he does not talk to the nurse, or the daughter may interrupt just as the nurse is about to receive important patient care information from the father. These maneuvers by family members keep the family functioning as it is. Because of this organized and repetitive sequence of interactions, families are quite resistant to change.

There are a number of norms that many families share. A common one is that anger is not expressed directly. One community health nurse remarked that although a family that she saw twice a week seemed to be seething underneath with rage, its members were unable to examine with her what might be causing the anger. Clearly a norm in this family was, "Don't express anger directly." When disagreement began in one family, the nurse noticed that general family uneasiness increased, and that the daughter always changed the subject. In this family, the daughter's behavior assisted the family to reestablish homeostasis.

When working with families, you have to decide whether you feel able to assist the family to show its feelings more directly. At times you may prefer to continue your work in an atmosphere of seething and hidden emotions. At other times, you may feel comfortable attempting to help the family express its anger more directly. In order to do so, you will probably need to seek guidance from a nurse who is more experienced and comfortable with working with family communication barriers.

Critical Events

Finding out about critical family events can give you a feel for what stresses the family is operating under as well as for what strengths the family has. Once you are aware of the stresses and strains the family is subject to, you may be more realistic about how influential you can be in changing or motivating a client or family. Such an examination will also give you clues about how to act to decrease further stress, and about how to support family members in their healthy coping attempts. In the family context, coping attempts can include all the ways in which family members pay attention to, make sense of, and respond to information in their internal and external environment. Adequate coping responses include the ability to vary behavior depending on environmental demands, the ability to problem-solve, and the ability to change behavior to meet the criteria of self and significant others (Coelho, 1974).

To determine whether a family is coping successfully, you must first assess its sources of stress. One source may lie in changes outside the family. War, recession, holidays, or weather changes, and neighborhood renovation or destruction are examples of some sources of potential stress that a family can encounter in areas outside the family.

Changes in the parents' own parents' (family of origin) health or behavior can create stress in a family. If an identified patient's favorite grandmother dies, or if a new mother quarrels with her own mother about how to care for her infant, family stress increases.

If someone enters or leaves the nuclear family, stress is increased. Examples of such stress-producing events include when a grandmother comes to live with a family, when a boarder is taken in, when a daughter gets married, or when a husband and father dies.

Biological changes in a family member can create stress for the family too. Such changes could include when a child reaches adolescence, when a mother starts menopause, when a father develops cancer, when a wife is diagnosed as having multiple sclerosis, or when a son develops symptoms of an ulcer.

Social and economic changes can also place increased pressures on a family. When a child starts kindergarten or college, when a family moves, when a father or husband gets or loses a job, when a family member starts to drink or take drugs excessively, the family is likely to experience increased stress. It is also important to assess the involvement of family members in social activities as a family, as separate people, and as members of the community. A family that shares some family activities, that allows its members to have individual activities, and that has community support from friends, clergy, and clubs or organizations will be more flexible and better able to handle stress than a family that does not have these alternative supports. Changes in vacation schedules can also influence family functioning. How the family uses or is prevented from using community resources such as schools and health agencies can also be assessed as to their influence on family functioning.

It is important to realize that what is stressful for one family may not be stressful for another. However, in general, if a family has experienced several of these critical events within the period of a year, it is probably in a state of severe stress.

In trying to assess critical events, try to evaluate the effect of these events on family relationships. Do family members pull closer together when they are under stress? Sometimes a crisis will bring family members together to work out a solution whereas their usual pattern of behavior is to withdraw from one another. Once the crisis is over, they may pull apart again and resume their individual interests. Do family members pull apart, go their own way, seem to run around in circles, or exaggerate their withdrawal from one another? Sometimes a crisis will appear to pull a family apart; once the crisis is over, exaggerated withdrawal from each other and attempts to get out of one another's way will cease. Do family members try to get rid of the upsetting family member? Sometimes the family seems to tire of dealing with a psychotic teenager, a confused grandparent, or a husband who has severely debilitating multiple sclerosis. Once the decision is made to send the teenager to a psychiatric facility, the grandmother to a nursing home, or the husband to an extended care facility, the crisis is resolved. Then again, if the decision was made without careful consideration, another crisis may arise as the family's level of guilt and anxiety increases. Does the family seem to show no reaction to the event? Some families might easily cope with a child's entering school, while others may not. Some families may deny that the event even occurred. Does the family seem to be blaming one family member for a change that is not necessarily anyone's fault? Sometimes families choose one family member to be the scapegoat for the family; when a crisis occurs, that person is blamed and berated for all that has happened. Sometimes the family might try to give the role of scapegoat to you. The members of other families may try to cope with family changes by denying the change, by trying to explain away the change, by starting a fight with another family member or with you, or by becoming depressed. It is also useful to attempt to evaluate the success level of the family's coping attempts. Some measures of unsuccessful coping attempts by family members may be expressing anger inappropriately, worrying about trivial events, wrangling over the same issue continuously, and putting each other down rather than problem-solving. Some measures of successful coping attempts may be accepting change, taking individual responsibility for behavior and decisions, being willing to meet obligations, being able to consider others' needs, and being able to discuss family problems objectively and reasonably. A first step that you may take in helping a family to cope better is to assess its ability to cope successfully or unsuccessfully with stress.

Roles

When two people marry, they bring with them to the marriage modes of behaving that they learned from their own parents. If a wife was her mother's helper, she may try to get her husband and children to cast her in the role of helpgiver. If a husband was picked on by his parents and siblings, he may try to get his wife and kids to pick on him too. This role is called the scapegoat role. If a wife broke up arguments between her own parents, she may continue to play the role of peacemaker in her own marriage. If a husband learned as a child that being funny and joking would decrease the tension between his mother and father, he may also try to play the role of joker with his wife and children. If a woman learned that she could never disagree with her parents without being directly or indirectly punished, she may try to always agree with her husband and children. Women who are anxious about their ability to mother or to assume roles other than that of mother may turn into smothering mothers who refuse to allow their children to be independent or to make decisions for themselves.

Because you grew up in a family, you have learned to play certain roles in family settings. You may feel most comfortable assuming any of the roles of helper, scapegoat, peacemaker, joker, agreer, or smothering mother. Superimposed on these possible learned family roles are the roles that you have been taught to assume during your nursing education. Some of these roles are those of teacher, information-giver, interpreter, and suggestion-giver. You may be more aware of assuming the latter roles, since replaying roles that were learned in one's own family often comes as second nature, and may be done unconsciously. It will be helpful to you in your work with families to try to become more aware of roles in which your own family cast you. Playing a role is really a two-way process. You cannot be cast in a role unless you agree to be, and others will not agree to cast you in that role unless they feel comfortable doing so or unless they do so out of desperation or need. You will meet families that try to cast you in roles that you do not wish to assume or that are familiar to you because you played that role in your own family. In either case, playing the role merely to please the family can create problems for you and the family.

It is fairly easy to see how roles such as that of smothering mother or joker are not useful ones for you to assume. It is less clear how your playing the roles of agreer or helper might be detrimental to a family. In general, you will be on the right track if you have at least some awareness of the roles that you are used to playing, and of the roles that families try to cast you in.

There are several roles that children usually play that you should watch out for. These are the roles of ally, messenger, peacemaker, interrupter, and substitute parent. In the ally role, the child is approached by one or both parents who attempt to persuade the child to side with him or her against the other parent. In the messenger role, the child is asked to carry messages back and forth between parents. In the peacemaker role, the child is asked (or learns that it is best) to stop disagreements between other family members. In the interrupter role, the child learns to interrupt family interactions in order to protect family members from confrontation and strife. In the substitute parent role, the child takes care of one or both of his or her parents.

Playing any one of these roles can be especially detrimental because all of them place undue responsibility on the child and do not allow him or her to focus sufficient attention on the important developmental tasks at hand. Because children who assume these roles cannot complete their normal developmental tasks, they will achieve a lower developmental level in their interpersonal relationships than children who do not have this burden.

Functional and Dysfunctional Family Relationships

There are characteristics of relationships that are generally considered to be *functional*. In general, functional family relationships are those where members are confident about their ability to relate; where communication is clear and direct, and feedback is asked for and responded to; where disagreement can occur without belittlement; where others are treated as (or as having the potential for being) masterful, sexual people; where behavioral limits are set and adhered to; and where others are allowed to be different and to have separate interests (Satir, 1964).

Signs that a family member is confident could be his or her speaking without hesitation, maintaining eye contact, or taking a risk by saying something that is unconventional or assertive. Direct and open communication is just that—there is no beating around the bush or speaking in such obscure terms that the other person thinks to himself, "Now, just what did she want me to do or say?" Asking for feedback means that the speaker asks the other(s), "Did you understand (agree, have some thoughts or feelings about) what I said?" The speaker can ask for feedback in nonverbal ways such as turning to the listener after speaking and raising the eyebrows as if to say, "What do you have to say about that?" Being receptive to feedback from others includes doing such things as listening when the other person responds, and responding in turn to what was said. Examples of disagreeing without belittling the other are when one family members says, "I don't agree, but you have a right to your opinion" or "That's not the way I see it, but it is another way to look at it." Treating the other as a masterful, sexual person means that each allows the other to be as independent, creative, and able to contribute to relationships as possible. An example of a functional relationship is allowing children and debilitated family members to state their opinions. Asking what other family members think, and holding family meetings to discuss family decisions are further examples of demonstrating respect for others. Assuming that the other can hear and understand even though at times he or she is confused, or including the other in family planning and deliberations although his or her body may be crippled or dysfunctional in some ways are other signs of functional family relationships. Demonstrating that the other is sexual and masterful might include a husband and wife discussing ways to continue their sexual relationship after one spouse has become physically disabled.

Anarchy would reign if parents let children or confused elders make crucial family decisions, or strike out and hurt other family members. In functional family relationships, limits are set on what behavior is permissible, and members adhere to these limits. Everyone knows where they stand and what behavior is acceptable or unacceptable. Allowing others to be different includes encouraging them to try new adventures or learning experiences, and deciding what family members will do together and what they will do separately. In functional families, there is some flexibility and there are attempts by family members to realign relationships with each other depending on current stresses. When crises occur, the family neither overprotects nor underprotects its members.

Dysfunctional family relationships are those where members have low self-esteem and, as a result, try to ward off feeling poorly about themselves by dominating, confusing, or belittling others. One or more family members may feel left out; give indirect and/or conflicting communicational messages; pay no attention to whether others hear or respond to their messages; get upset when others do respond to their messages; belittle others who disagree with them; view others as weak, asexual, or less effective than they are or can be; set limits on others' behavior and then permit the behavior to occur; and not allow others to be different or to decide what the family members will do together and separately (Satir, 1964; 1975). Dysfunctional families are quite rigid and seem to keep trying to use old methods of adaptation despite the fact that these old methods may not work anymore (Watzlawick, 1974). These families tend to become overly concerned with a symptom or behavior of one of its members or to completely ignore critical symptoms or behaviors.

Leadership

Family *leadership* can be viewed as a set of functions rather than as a position assumed by parents or adults only. As long as some family member provides this set of functions, leadership exists. Once accepted by the family, you can provide needed leadership functions and/or teach family members to assume leadership within the family. Some leadership functions that you can evaluate with the families that you see are being attentive to others' needs; supporting others; clarifying unclear communication; summarizing discussions; encouraging all family members to participate; and focusing on the task. Focusing on the task could include activities such as giving information, redirecting conversation back to an important topic, and helping family members to evaluate situations or decisions (Clark, 1977).

Leadership functions that do not help family functioning include continuing to discuss only one family member's needs or interests; taking sides in an argument; and dominating others.

Disruptions

Disruptions include any behaviors that interfere with the nurse and family meeting the goals of the visit. At times you may be the disruptive factor because you are anxious, fearful, guilt-ridden, or fatigued; your own feelings and needs can disrupt your work with a family when you are unaware of how they may be affecting your interventions. At other times, family members may be the disruptive factors. They may change the subject, refuse to comply with the agreed-upon goals, interrupt one another or you, arrive late, or leave early.

General Atmosphere

Every interpersonal encounter has an atmosphere. Whenever you visit a home or work with a client or family in an agency, you will immediately get a sense of welcome, mistrust, anxiety, competitiveness, hopelessness, depression, formality, or support. Being able to tune into the atmosphere of a home or of a visit can help you to determine how to approach a client or family.

Phases of Interaction

Interactions between people usually have a beginning, a middle, and an end. Each visit that you have with a family also has these three phases of beginning, middle, and end. At the beginning of a visit you can expect some anxiety to occur in yourself and in family members. There is usually a period of socialization and greeting, and then some uncertainty about how to proceed. The middle phase of a visit may be the time when tasks are accomplished. Anxiety may or may not be lower during this phase. The end of a visit is when anxiety may again increase, plans for the next visit are made, and social leave-taking occurs. See Figure 12-2 for a sample Family Observation and Assessment Guide.

HOW TO USE THE GUIDE

Just as each family visit is different, each family system is different. By using the Family Observation and Assessment Guide, you can become more aware of how family events affect family interaction. You will begin to recognize how seating arrangement, norms, and leadership can promote or interfere with clear communication. You will notice how family members play roles in the family and how these roles affect the larger family system.

Figure 12-2 Sample Family Observation and Assessment Guide

Nurse _Carolyn Clark_

Date _4/26_

Length of visit _1 hour_

Who is present: Mrs. R. (IP), Mr. R., Robin (age 12)

Seating arrangement:
first half hour:

Mrs. R. (IP) → Robin
↕
→ me ←
Mr. R. (in kitchen)

2nd half hour: me ←

Mrs. R.
↕
→ Robin

Anxiety levels:	low	moderate	high
Beginning of visit			✓
Middle of visit		✓	
End of visit			✓

Norms: Accept tea
No swearing in front of guests
No anger expressed openly

Critical events

Changes outside of the family (examples):

Changes in the family or origin (examples): grandmother died last year

Entrance or exit of family members (examples):

Biological changes (examples): Robin began menstruating last week
Mrs. R. was discharged from the hospital last week

Social changes (examples): Mr. R. lost his job last month

Figure 12-2 Sample Family Observation and Assessment Guide (*Continued*)

Apparent effect of changes on family relationships: *Role reversal; Mr. R. now takes care of household*

Ways in which family copes with changes: *Uses denial; feelings go underground and emerge as putdowns and angry outbursts*

Roles that family plays: (e.g., scapegoat, smothering mother, helper, joker, antagonizer, suggestions giver, interpreter, interrupter, ally, messenger, pacifier)

Mother: *antagonizer (complains about Mr. R's care of Lee)*

Father: *helper*

Child: *interrupter; messenger; scapegoat*

Child:

Child:

Nurse: *suggestion-giver*

Other:

How are these roles maintained? (examples): *Mother and father neutralize one another until disagreement occurs; then Robin interrupts or is blamed for how she is acting. Robin agrees to take messages to others. Nurse gives advice when asked.*

Family Relationships:

Functional	Dysfunctional
____ is confident example:	✓ fears being left out example: *Robin interrupts*
____ directly asks for help example:	✓ communication is indirect/conflicting example: *Mrs R. asks Robin to give messages to Mr. R. or talks about him, not to him.*
✓ asks for feedback example: *Mrs. R. asks Robin for Lee ideas.*	____ does not care if messages are received example:

Figure 12-2   Sample Family Observation and Assessment Guide (*Continued*)

_____ is receptive to feedback
      example:

__✓__ gets upset when receives feedback
      example: *Robin starts yelling when Mrs. R. disagrees with her.*

__✓__ disagrees without attacking
      example: *Mrs. R. disagrees with Robin.*

_____ disagrees with attack/diverts disagreement
      example:

_____ treats other as capable
      example:

__✓__ treats other as totally dependent/helpless
      example: *Mrs. R. says Mr. R. is "hopeless in the kitchen."*

_____ sets limits and sticks to them
      example:

__✓__ does not maintain set limits
      example: *Mrs. R. tells Robin not to touch candy, then lets her have 3 pieces.*

_____ allows others to be different
      example:

_____ does not allow others to be different
      example:

_____ has relationships with others in the community
      example:

__✓__ is isolated from community supports
      example: *Mrs. R. says the family "does everything together."*

Leadership:

        Individual members

        Family as a whole

_____ is attentive to others' needs
      example:

_____ achieves a balance between accomplishing a task and having fun
      example:

_____ supports others
      example:

_____ has some form of leadership
      example:

__✓__ focuses on self only
      example: *Mrs. R. talks mostly about her body and eating patterns.*

_____ members speak clearly and openly to each other about needs and wants
      example:

_____ takes sides
      example:

_____ members neither shy away from nor provoke conflict
      example:

Figure 12-2   Sample Family Observation and Assessment Guide (*Continued*)

✓ dominates other
     example: *Mrs. R. tries to prevent Mr. R. from answering my questions.*

✓ clarifies unclear communication
     example: *I try to clarify Mrs. R's comments.*

_____ summarizes discussion
     example:

_____ encourages quiet members to participate
     example:

_____ focuses on task
     example:

Disruptions:

Who disrupts the visit and how: *Robin interrupts others' comments*

General atmosphere (e.g., formal, cooperative, informal, supportive, competitive, hostile):
informal and competitive

Phases:

What kinds of behaviors are evident at the beginning of the visit: *Mrs. R. talks very fast; Robin interrupts alot.*

What kinds of behaviors are evident at the middle of the visit: *Mr. R. goes into the garage; Mrs. R. talks more slowly; Robin interrupts less.*

What kinds of behaviors are evident at the end of the visit: *Mrs. R. talks faster and seems to want me to stay longer.*

Nursing diagnoses:

1. *unresolved grief over grandmother*
2. *inability of mother to re-enter family role*
3. *role reversal of marital pair*
4. *changes in body image for Robin*
5. *indirect family communication patterns*

You might want to use the guide in order to make an initial assessment of the mental health aspects of family functioning. You could refer to the guide prior to your meeting with the family. It is not suggested that you have the guide in view because, if family members see it, they may think that you are observing them under a microscope. You may wish to jot down key questions that you wish to ask in order to make your assessment, or you may wish to devise your own symbol system to remind you of behavior that you should watch for. If any family member asks you what you are writing, simply say, "I want to write down what happens so I don't forget." You can fill in the guide soon after you complete the visit by referring to your notes; or, if you prefer not to take notes while you are with the family, write your comments down as soon as you finish the visit because recall diminishes rapidly and you will soon forget important points.

The guide can also be used at crucial points with a family you are seeing on a long-term basis; the information you glean could help you to see changes that are occurring over time in the family system.

You might also use the guide to compare several different families with whom you are working. By gathering the kind of information asked for in the guide, you can begin to see how family systems differ from and resemble one another.

By using the guide to gather information, you will begin to see how to intervene in family systems. The guide is a beginning tool, and you will probably require further supervision or consultation from a more skilled nurse about what interventions may be useful.

Although you as a nurse must try not to become part of the family system, your behavior will affect what happens within the family. Because this is so, it is important to study how your behavior changes with different families and to speculate on why this is so. For example, the roles that you assume in one family may be directly evoked by that family, but not by other families. Since nurses are expected to promote healthy behaviors in families, you would want to assess and intervene in your own behavior if it seems to be promoting dysfunctional relationships within one or more families.

SUMMARY

The Family Observation and Assessment Guide can help you to become aware of ways in which the family tries to draw you into becoming part of its way of functioning. The guide can help you to identify both functional and dysfunctional relationships that occur in families that you see. The information that you glean from the guide can help you to be more effective in family teaching, counseling, and communication.

There are at least eleven areas of family functioning that can be observed and assessed: who is present during the visit, seating arrangement, anxiety levels, family norms, critical events, family roles, functional and dysfunctional relationships, leadership, disruptions, general atmosphere, and phases of interaction.

PRACTICE EXERCISES

Use the Family Observation and Assessment Guide to assess two families that you have visited or are about to visit. Try to make comparisons between the two families regarding family norms, roles, relationships, and leadership. Compare the information that you have obtained with knowledge that you already have about your own family.

REVIEW

Listing

List eleven areas of family assessment and write down an example for each assessment based on your observations of a family.

1 _____

Example:

2 _____

Example:

3 _____

Example:

4 _____

Example:

5 _____

Example:

6 _____

Example:

7 _____

Example:

8 _____

Example:

9 _____

Example:

10 _____

Example:

11 _____

Example:

REFERENCES

Clark, Carolyn Chambers. 1977. *The nurse as group leader.* New York: Springer.

Coelho, George V., ed. 1974. *Coping and adaptation.* New York: Springer.

Group for Advancement of Psychiatry. 1973. *Assessment of sexual function: a guide to interviewing.* New York: Aronson.

Hall, Joanne, and Weaver, Barbara R. 1974. *Nursing of families in crisis.* Philadelphia: Lippincott.

Noland, Robert L. 1971. *Counseling parents of the ill and the handicapped.* Springfield, Ill. Thomas.

Satir, Virginia. 1964. *Conjoint family therapy.* Palo Alto: Science and Behavior Books.

_____ et al. 1975. *Helping families to change.* New York: Aronson.

Watzlawick, Paul, et al. 1974. *Change.* New York: Norton.

Chapter 13

Mental Health Consultation

LEARNING OBJECTIVES

When you finish this chapter, you should be able to:

- Give an example of one sign that mental health nursing consultation is needed
- List several common reactions to mental health nursing consultation
- Define *theme*
- Tell why being able to identify themes is a useful skill

At times you may experience severe discomfort when working with a client or family. It may not be clear to you at the time what the source of the discomfort is. You may have reviewed your sources of anxiety, attempted to complete a process recording for the client, and/or used the Family Observation and Assessment Guide. When none of these procedures serves to decrease your discomfort, you may decide that it is time to turn to a mental health nursing consultant. Your increasing discomfort when working with a client may be a signal that consultation is needed.

MENTAL HEALTH CONSULTATION

Mental health consultation is an interpersonal process in which you work with an expert, such as a mental health nursing specialist, to define and solve a client or family problem. Many mental health nursing consultants are not members of agency staffs. They are called in on a contract or case basis. When one or more community health nurses experience anxiety about working with a client, consultation may be the solution. Consultation is not psychotherapy or psychoanalysis, and should focus on the nurse-client relationship. Since the consultant has no real authority over you, his or her expertise and skill in relating to you will form the basis of the consultant-consultee relationship, and will affect whether you will eventually implement the suggestions that are made to you during a consultation session.

If you have never worked with a consultant, you may have some reservations about the idea. You may be anxious and on the defensive. This is to be expected since the consultation process is a new and unfamiliar situation. You may find some of the following thoughts crossing your mind when the idea of a mental health nursing consultant is suggested to you:

"I don't have *that* many problems!"
"I don't need psychotherapy."
"Perhaps the consultant can just take over the whole case."
"I must not be very competent if I need consultation."
"I don't have any psychiatric clients, so why would I need mental health nursing consultation?"
"I don't have time to sit down with a consultant."
"Consultants may know a lot of theory, but they don't know much about actually working with clients."

All of these reactions occur fairly frequently prior to consultation and are no cause for alarm. However, if these thoughts continue to recur, it may be wise for you to bring them up for discussion with the consultant. You are within your rights to also ask the consultant to tell you about his or her training to be a consultant and why he or she wishes to work with your agency. If you continue to feel ambivalent, you may wish to seek out a different consultant.

Not all consultants work in the same way. The more complicated the interpersonal problem between you and your client, the longer it will often take for you and the consultant to unravel the problem and decide on an intervention. Sometimes consultants work with groups of nurses. Group consultation can be effective for a number of reasons:

1 If several community health nurses work with one client or family, a group discussion allows them to share their information with each other.

2 Group discussion can provide support. It may be reassuring for you to hear that others (including some consultants) are also anxious, frustrated, or whatever when working with certain clients.

3 Continuity of care can be promoted through group problem solving.

4 You can learn how to review others' work and to assist them in identifying problems by observing and imitating comments that are made by the consultant.

5 If the supervisor or administrator of the agency is included in group consultation, there is a greater chance for communication channels in the agency to be opened up.

A group consultation on one client or family can rarely be accomplished in a session shorter than an hour and one-half. Individual consultations may be shorter if the interpersonal problem is uncomplicated and if the consultee has some grasp of what the problem is. Most of the time, you may be quite unclear about what the problem is.

Whether you participate in individual or group consultation sessions, the process will be the same, and follows the flow of any problem-solving situation. First, the problem is defined. Second, facts and hunches about the problem are discussed or analyzed. Third, interventions and solutions that have already been tried are examined. Fourth, alternate solutions or hypotheses are listed. Fifth, a solution is chosen and then tried out. Sixth, a way to evaluate the result is found.

Since it is not always clear what the problem is, you may wish to use a form similar to the one in Figure 13-1 to help you to focus on the client and family. This guide will be used extensively in the "Case Consultations for Discussion"; therefore, only its format is presented here.

HOW TO USE THE MENTAL HEALTH CONSULTATION GUIDE

You can use the Mental Health Consultation Guide in a number of ways. The material in Part A can be identified by you prior to an upcoming visit with a client and presented to the consultant who can then assist you to plan interventions. A variation on this approach is to have the consultant make the visit with you (after a preconference to evaluate the information acquired in Part A) for the purpose of assessing your interaction with clients or so that he or she can role model interventions with the specific family. This approach requires you to have established a relationship of trust and collaboration with the consultant and to feel free to learn and/or experiment without being anxious and competing with the consultant about who can deal most effectively with the family.

Another way to use the guide is for group consultation. You present the data in Part A to a group of your peers and the consultant. Problems and goals are then identified by the group with assistance from the consultant. At times themes or problems may not be clear to you. A *theme* is a recurrent happening

Figure 13-1 Mental Health Consultation Guide

Part A

---

1 Family members and their problems
  a Who lives in the house?
  b What are the medical problems of each member?
  c What are the interpersonal or communication problems of each member?
  d What are the social and/or occupational problems of each member?
2 Reason for presenting this case for consultation
  a Do you need help in clarifying what is going on between you and the family?
  b Do you think that the consultant needs to visit the family with you?
  c Do you need help in deciding which family members need your services?
  d Do you think that the problems are beyond the scope of your skills, thereby requir-
      ing the assistance of another professional? If so, who do you think would provide the
      most help?

Part B

---

3 Problems, goals, and suggested interventions identified through consultation

  a _____

  b _____

  c _____

  d _____

Part C

---

4 Evaluation
  a How did the suggested interventions seem to work?
  b In what ways was consultation helpful? unhelpful?
  c What suggestions can you make for future consultations?

---

or message. Often a visit will have only one theme. The client may tell you
through words and actions the same message using different words and actions
each time. Feelings are often themes, as are thoughts the client implies or verbal-
izes to you. Some common themes that clients may direct toward you are:

I'm helpless (hopeless).
I will resist you.
I'm afraid.
I'm anxious (angry).
I feel guilty.
I am bad.
I'm (he's or she's) out of control.

I can't wait for gratification.
I can't decide.
I'm in charge here.
I'm omnipotent.

Being able to identify themes in your interactions with clients will be helpful to you. First, themes are often clearer indicants of how clients view themselves and others than isolated phrases or answers to questions are. Themes can often be inferred from nonverbal communication such as tone of voice and activity (or lack of it). Second, themes will give you clues about your own reactions to clients and your blindspots. Everyone has blindspots or areas of interpersonal sensitivity that they are not totally aware of. These areas can cause you to become defensive and not listen to the client. By trying to become attuned to your own blindspots, you will become more attuned to what is happening in the relationship between you and your client. Some themes that you may recognize in your interactions with clients are:

I want to protect you.
I'm bad (incompetent) if you don't improve.
You're (I'm) hopeless/helpless.
I'm anxious (angry).
I feel guilty.
You're not motivated.

If you react with some clients in your characteristic way, you may immediately find yourself in a blow-up situation. For example, if both you and the client insist on being in charge, you will precipitate a confrontation. Whereas, if you feel comfortable taking charge and the client feels helpless, in the short run your relationship will seem smooth; however, your taking charge may lead to difficulties later on when you have established the client's dependency but then wish him or her to shift gears and somehow know how to be independent. The mental health consultant may wish to use the same form that the community health nurse uses to present to the consultant, or the consultant may wish to take process notes of the discussion for his or her own use.

It is not unusual for themes to emerge in a group consultation session that mirror problems that are occurring in the nurse's work with clients. Figure 13-2 shows a sample recording made by the mental health nursing consultant where this happened.

It is preferable that an evaluation be conducted after each consultation. The evaluation should include an examination of how the suggested interventions changed (or did not change) the nurse-client relationship problem as well as an effort to identify what is helpful and unhelpful to the consultee-consultant relationship.

Figure 13-2   Team Conference Notes Prepared by the Consultant

---

Oscar A, a 20-year-old with multiple congenital deformities

DISCUSSION

A discussion among the visiting nurses, members of the homemaker staff, welfare service worker, and physical therapist raised the following issues:

1 Oscar probably has profound self- and body image difficulties due to his 20-year history of physical debilitation and inexperience in interpersonal situations.

2 There is mounting resentment in Oscar's sister, Patty, because she has been asked to assume more of his care since their mother left the family. This loss of a family member has probably created an imbalance in the family that it seems to have resolved by trying to force Patty, age 17, into the role of surrogate wife-mother. Another example of the family's unsuccessful coping is Mr. A's help-rejecting, complaining way of relating with health workers. Mr. A has solicited the help of many health workers, but thus far has refused to take any of their advice.

3 The family appears to have unresolved grief over the following experiences: Oscar's loss of body control; the loss of the wife-mother; the father's increasing physical withdrawal (from a situation that he may regard as intolerable); and the threatened loss of Patty who refuses to take on the surrogate wife-mother role.

4 An overriding issue of concern is the high degree of emotional involvement of the health workers. There seem to be strong feelings of frustration, anger, helplessness, and hopelessness present in many members of the health team involved with the A family. Such reactions are not unexpected because of their great efforts to help this family and the kinds of feelings a help-rejecting family is likely to evoke in those who offer to help it. The feelings of the staff perhaps need further consideration and separating out so that the likelihood of angry interchanges with the family and/or withdrawal from it is minimized.

5 There was evidence of conflict among staff members when they were discussing goals of treatment for the A family. Although there was a complaint that family members are passively resistant without directly rejecting advice, there is some indication that staff members are hesitant to present their thoughts and feelings about care to the family in a direct manner. Indirect communication from family to health caregivers and vice versa is probably encouraging a vicious cycle of frustration and helplessness.

6 Perhaps due to the difficulty of viewing the family as a system, several participants cast family members in the roles of "good" or "noncooperative" rather than seeing each member of the family as cooperating on some level with one another to produce a family system that maintains homeostasis.

INTERVENTIONS SUGGESTED BY THE CONSULTANT

1 Try to view families as systems. Begin to ask questions such as: "What purpose is this behavior serving in the family now?" "Who else allows this kind of behavior to continue in the family?" "How am I supporting or disrupting the family's coping attempts?"

2 Since Oscar probably feels very helpless in the family, he may be using passive resistance as the only method of controlling what happens to him. Suggest that Oscar reframe his behavior by making comments to him such as, "Gee, you really have a lot of power in this house. Just by not agreeing, you can control what the family does." Another method that might decrease Oscar's probable feelings of helplessness and powerlessness as well as increase his ability to relate interpersonally is to structure a one-to-one

Figure 13-2 Team Conference Notes Prepared by the Consultant (*Continued*)

relationship for him with another person. The most likely candidates for his partner in this relationship are the homemaker who seems to be able to relate positively to Oscar, or the male sibling whom Oscar can perhaps relate to as "we're the young men in this family." Whoever agrees to take on this relationship will probably require support and direction from supervisory staff at the agency.

3 Suggest that the helpgivers begin an ongoing discussion to determine the limits of care for families. Part of this discussion would include a clarification of third-party payment limits, but would also include professional nursing judgments about goals for treatment, how much the family is to be included in setting these goals, and whether or not families are to be told from the first visit that care is limited to x number of visits with the option to extend care upon joint evaluation and agreement.

4 Suggest that a joint conference be held by health team members and the family to discuss further plans for the family.

5 Agree with the suggestion of the welfare worker to contact the school social worker about taking some family pressure off Patty and/or providing some support for her so that she need not leave the family precipitously.

GROUND DYNAMICS OF THE CONSULTATION

It was noted that the discussion by the health team followed somewhat the same course as reported visits to the A family; i.e., there was help-rejecting behavior, complaining, indirect communication, and conflict evident in the health workers' interactions with one another and with the consultant.

Until you have experience working with a consultant, the process of identifying problems may seem somewhat mysterious. If you are able to work with a consultant, you could be wise to ask for clarification whenever you do not understand any impressions or suggestions that the consultant presents.

SUMMARY

Mental health consultation is an interpersonal process in which you work with an expert to define and solve a client or family problem. It is not unusual for people to initially resist the idea of consultation, but the process can provide opportunities for sharing information, offering support, promoting continuity of care, learning how to review others' work, and opening up channels of communication within an agency.

PRACTICE EXERCISES

1 Identify several clients who would benefit from your seeking mental health nursing consultation.

2 Devise a way to obtain the needed consultation.

REVIEW

Definition

Define theme.

_____

Listing

1 Give an example of one sign that mental health consultation is needed.

_____

2 List two reasons why being able to identify themes is a useful skill.

_____

_____

3 List several common reactions to mental health nursing consultation.

_____

_____

_____

_____

REFERENCES

Caplan, G. 1959. *Concepts of mental health and consultation.* USDHEW, PHS and Mental Health Administration. Maternal and Child Health Service. PHS Publication #2072.

Caplan, G. 1970. *The theory and practice of mental health consultation.* New York: Basic Books.

Clark, Carolyn Chambers. 1976. Psychiatric Mental Health Consultation with Nurses. Paper read at New York State Nurses' Association Convention, 11–15 October 1976, at Grossinger, New York.

Deloughery, G. et al. 1971. *Consultation and community organization in community mental health nursing.* Baltimore: Williams and Wilkins.

Forti, T. 1970. Mental health consultation: one key to planned change. *Nursing Outlook* 18, 7:42–45.

Mouw, M., and Haylett, C. 1975. Community mental health nursing and consultation. In *Contemporary community nursing*, ed. B. Spradley, pp. Boston: Little, Brown.

Part Three

Case Consultations and Discussions

The purpose of this part is to illustrate, through the use of case consultations and discussions, the theories, concepts, and guides presented in the first two parts of this book. As a result, the applicability of core mental health concepts and interventions to your work with clients will hopefully become evident. It may be helpful for you to go through these cases and discussions with another nurse, group of peers, or supervisor and to consider how specific problems and interventions were identified.

Case 1
Mr. Caldron Has Arthritis

FAMILY MEMBERS AND THEIR PROBLEMS

Mr. Caldron, 28, has had rheumatoid arthritis since he was 18. One month ago he had a total replacement of his right hip. He lives in an apartment that is connected to his parents' home. His mother is described by the community health nurse as superficially gracious, but more interested in the infants she babysits with than in anything else. Mr. Caldron's father does all his son's physical care including helping him to bed and to the toilet, but rarely talks to him or to the nurse. Mr. Caldron was married for 1 year but his wife left him 1 year ago; he seems uncomfortable with this topic and has not discussed the circumstances surrounding the break up of his marriage with the nurse, except to question whether his wife's leaving may have been an attempt to punish him. Mr. Caldron takes no responsibility for his activities of daily living. Although physiotherapy has been recommended, the family has been unable to plan for one treatment to take place.

REASON FOR CONSULTATION

The community health nurse expressed a need for suggestions about how to talk more freely with Mr. Caldron and for suggestions about how to involve family members in talking with one another. The nurse also suggested that the consultant visit the home with her and evaluate communication difficulties and nursing interventions.

PROBLEMS AND INTERVENTIONS IDENTIFIED
THROUGH CONSULTATION

The consultant and community health nurse agreed to visit the Caldron home together. Following the visit, the following problems were discussed and the following interventions were agreed upon.

Problems	Interventions
1 Asking questions that can be answered with a "yes" or a "no."	1 Ask questions such as, "What else was going on then?" "Who was there?" "What was said?" "What did you think (feel) then?"

2 Unresolved grief related to Mr. Caldron's loss of his body function and wife.

2 Suggest by word and action that such losses can be discussed.
   a Pick up and explore any comment that is related to the client's loss or grief; e.g., make statements such as, "Tell me more about that" "It may be difficult to talk about this, but it can be helpful to you."
   b Maintain eye contact with the client when he talks about his losses.
   c Allow the client to break silences and/or encourage him to go on with the topic being discussed.

3 Lack of interpersonal support among family members.

3 Teach family members how to support one another.
   a Encourage the family to sit down with the community health nurse and focus on a circumscribed task such as planning a visit to the physiotherapist.
   b Do not allow family members to speak for one another or to berate one another without your trying to intervene by demonstrating other ways for them to relate.

4 Tendency of Mr. Caldron to negate the validity of his thoughts and feelings; e.g., he makes comments such as, "That's stupid of me" or "I guess I don't know any better."

4 Bolster self-esteem of Mr. Caldron.
   a Encourage the client to examine his self-evaluations, e.g., ask questions such as "What do you think is stupid about that?" or "Where did you get the idea that you don't know any better?"
   b Teach Mr. Caldron to speak for himself with other family members.

5 Client dependency.

5 Encourage client independence.
   a Ask for the client's thoughts and feelings.
   b Comment on constructive solutions or ideas, e.g., "That seem reasonable to me."
   c Gradually increase the difficulty of problem-solving tasks for the client.

EVALUATION

Two weeks after the joint consultant-nurse home visit, the community health nurse wrote the following evaluation:

> I am beginning to reformulate my questions to Mr. Caldron so that he has to do more thinking and talking. I am working to use silence more effectively, but still get anxious when silences last more than a minute. I have been unable to get the whole family to sit down to talk with me about a physiotherapy appointment for Mr. Caldron, but I noticed that his father made a spontaneous comment to him about how he walks better now. I am beginning to see how the family system works, and to view Mrs. Caldron as less of a bad mother.
>
> The consultation helped me to step back and take an objective look at the family and at how I was relating to the identified patient and to other family members as well. The home visit would have been more helpful if the consultant had demonstrated effective one-to-one and nurse-to-family communication techniques for me to observe. I suggest that the consultant and community health nurse work out their agenda prior to the visit, and decide if the consultant will function as an observer or as a role model.

Case 2

Patty Rodriguez Has Diabetes

FAMILY MEMBERS AND THEIR PROBLEMS

Patty, age 15, has juvenile diabetes. She has three younger siblings. She does not give herself her own insulin and will not stay on her diet. She was hospitalized recently for acidosis. Patty does not seem to have accepted that she has diabetes, and refuses to tell other people that she does. Patty's mother tells everyone about Patty's condition and makes arrangements for her. Patty stays out late at night and then misses breakfast because she sleeps late. Patty's father has been out of work for 2 years.

REASON FOR CONSULTATION

The community health nurse expressed concern about Patty, and some irritation with Patty's parents. She requested suggestions for helping Patty to become more responsible.

PROBLEMS AND INTERVENTIONS IDENTIFIED
THROUGH CONSULTATION

The consultant summarized the following problems and suggested the following interventions following a group consultation:

Problems	Interventions
1 Patty's unresolved grief.	1 a Help Patty to begin talking about her feelings about having diabetes. b Suggest that Patty join a group for teenagers who have diabetes where she could discuss her thoughts and feelings about having diabetes with her peers.
2 Triangling of nurse into family system.	2 Ask nurse to examine her own reaction of wanting to protect Patty. a Support Patty's relationship with the school nurse as a female role model who might encourage her independence. b Provide support for Patty's father who is grieving the loss of his job and for her mother who may resent her husband's unemployment and her daughter's seeming nonresponse to her.

3 Patty's inability to stay on her diet.

3 Help family to develop a behavioral contract; e.g., Patty can stay out late 1 night whenever she follows her diet for 1 day; Patty's father could monitor this and the nurse will talk with Patty's mother for 15 minutes whenever she does not nag her daughter.

EVALUATION

One month after the consultation, the community health nurse wrote the following evaluation:

> Patty is beginning to talk with the school nurse about her thoughts and feelings about having diabetes. She has agreed to join a group for teenagers who have diabetes. I feel less in the middle between Patty and her parents and have developed a better relationship with Patty's mother. Patty and her family are working with me to develop a behavioral contract to help her to stay on her diet. Next, I plan to work on one with Patty to help her to give herself her own insulin.
>
> The consultation helped me to see how I had been triangled in by the family. I also benefited from hearing the supportive comments of the other nurses.

Case 3

Mr. Washington Has a Colostomy

FAMILY MEMBERS AND THEIR PROBLEMS

Mr. Washington has been out of the hospital for 1 month following a temporary colostomy for diverticulitis. During his hospital stay, he had the following complications: congestive heart failure, rectal abcesses, anemia, and iritis. Since arriving home, he has abdicated the care of his colostomy to his wife who had some experience caring for her own mother. The community health nurse expressed concern about whether a more concerted effort should be made to teach the client how to care for his colostomy.

REASON FOR CONSULTATION

During a conference prior to the joint home visit of the nurse and consultant, the following questions were raised for clarification.

What is the status of the client's iritis? (It was decided that the nurse would check with the physician in order to ascertain this.)

When will the colostomy be closed? If soon, is it necessary to teach the client how to care for it?

What is the purpose of the wife's caring for the colostomy? Does this arrangement help the couple to cope more effectively?

What are the client's feelings about the colostomy and the complications that occurred during his hospitalization?

THE HOME VISIT

During the home visit, Mr. Washington seemed anxious and appeared to have some difficulty hearing what was being said. This may have been a function of his anxiety since he only had this difficulty when asked about his feelings. His denial of the situation was also evident; during the first half of the visit, he maintained that he had no thoughts or feelings about his life situation. As the visit progressed, he became more verbal and with encouragement was able to participate in cleaning the stoma and stated that he would learn how to dilate it if necessary. It seemed to be a useful intervention with this client to talk about the size, color, quantity of fecal material, etc. As the consultant talked about these matters, the community health nurse removed the colostomy bag. While the consultant continued to talk, the client became curious and began to look at the stoma, and, finally, with encouragement, he began to cleanse the area.

According to the community health nurse, this was the first visit during which the wife was not in the room at all times. Her absence may have been a factor in Mr. Washington's ability to move out of the denial stage of grief. Since it is difficult to tell when a person will resolve his or her grief, it is also difficult to know when that person will be receptive to teaching; the client will not learn if he or she is totally denying the situation.

At one point, the wife entered the bedroom for a few minutes, but seemed extremely uncomfortable, especially when she was asked questions. She stated that she did her husband's colostomy care because he had been so weak upon his return from the hospital, and also because she did not mind doing it. The consultant stated that Mr. Washington was stronger now and suggested that perhaps he could assist with his own care.

PROBLEMS AND INTERVENTIONS IDENTIFIED THROUGH CONSULTATION

Following the visit, the consultant and community health nurse agreed upon the following interventions for the identified problems.

Problems	Intervention
1 Denial of situation by the client.	1 Continue to encourage the client to view and learn about the colostomy especially if the colostomy is permanent.
2 Client dependency/communication.	2 a Talk with the wife in order to ascertain the reason behind her need to care for her husband. b Decide whether it is important or not for the client to help care for the colostomy; e.g., check with the doctor about his or her plans for the client, talk with both husband and wife about their wishes. c Help the couple to develop a behavioral contract and/or a reinforcement schedule as necessary.
3 Client anxiety.	3 Using facilitative questions, encourage the client to describe his thoughts and feelings.

EVALUATION

After the consultation, the community health nurse wrote the following evaluation:

Having the consultant accompany me to the home provided support by allowing me to see that the client's reaction occurred independent of my care. When the consultant first arrived, he was no more helpful or verbal than he had been with me.

The doctor confirmed that the colostomy would remain in place for at least 2 more months, so I have begun to teach Mr. and Mrs. Washington how to share care of the colostomy. I also spend time talking with each of them about their thoughts and feelings; this seems to have decreased anxiety as evidenced by Mr. Washington's ability to describe his thoughts and feelings, and Mrs. Washington's willingness to allow her husband to help with some of his care.

Case 4
Mr. Jotter Is Depressed/Suicidal

FAMILY MEMBERS AND THEIR PROBLEMS

Mr. Jotter has recently moved in with his daughter's family, the Tinleys, following his discharge from the hospital after a right femoral embolectomy. Mr. Jotter has been more depressed, and has become more physically dependent on his daughter since he has become increasingly debilitated. Mrs. Tinley reports feeling pressure from her father and her brothers and sisters to care for Mr. Jotter and not to place him in a nursing home. Mrs. Tinley complains of feeling guilty and helpless. Her husband works 12 to 14 hours a day and leaves the care of their two young sons and her father to her.

The community health nurse identified the following family dynamics. Mr. Jotter and his daughter talk to the nurse, but not to each other. Mrs. Tinley answers for Mr. Jotter and disparages what he says. Family norms are that family members cannot express their feelings directly to each other, and that Mrs. Tinley is more knowledgeable than her father. The community health nurse has taken on the role of supporter, while he characterizes Mrs. Tinley's role as that of martyr.

Changes in the family system include Mr. Jotter's coming to live with his daughter, and the upcoming entrance of Mrs. Tinley's youngest child into school.

REASON FOR CONSULTATION

The community health nurse asked for help in evaluating the depression level and possible suicide level of Mr. Jotter. He recalled that Mr. Jotter made several offhand comments such as, "I'm not sure it's worth it" and "Life doesn't mean much any more." He also requested help in making family communication clearer.

PROBLEMS AND INTERVENTIONS IDENTIFIED THROUGH CONSULTATION

In an individual consultation session, the following problems and interventions were identified.

Problems	Interventions
1 Evaluate Mr. Jotter's depression/suicide level.	**1** Ask the client whether he has thought about killing himself.
	a If so, ask what his plan is.
	b Encourage him to share his feelings with the nurse and with other family members.
	c Be sure he knows his family must be told about his plans for suicide.
	d Work out an alternate way for the client to handle his suicidal impulses; e.g., talk with the nurse or his daughter, call suicide prevention center.
	e Talk with the daughter and teach her about suicide clues, and how to respond when (if) her father threatens suicide.
2 Mrs. Tinley's conflict.	**2** Decrease the client's feelings of conflict.
	a Assist Mrs. Tinley to examine the pros and cons of keeping her father in her home.
	b Encourage her to share her feelings with her father.
3 Family communication.	**3** Promote family interaction.
	a Encourage "I" messages not "you" (blaming) messages.
	b Encourage activities where grandfather and grandchildren participate together.
	c Ask the client to talk directly to his daughter (and vice versa) rather than talking to the nurse.

EVALUATION

The community health nurse wrote the following evaluation 3 weeks after the consultation:

> Mr. Jotter denied having any suicidal thoughts. Before I had time to talk with Mrs. Tinley about this, Mr. Jotter made a suicidal threat. He picked up an ax in the garage and said he was going to end it all. His daughter evidently told him to stop being silly. That night he locked himself in the bathroom and cut his throat (superficially) with a razor blade. Mrs. Tinley immediately called an ambulance and had him hospitalized in the county psychiatric hospital.
>
> I felt guilty and upset. I asked the consultant to call a staff meeting so that we could discuss the event. After the meeting, I felt better. I guess the family concealed some information from me, or perhaps hospitalizing Mr. Jotter was the only way the family could resolve its conflict and guilt. Next time I will teach family members how to deal more effectively with suicidal thoughts and attempts. I think I learned a lot from this episode.

Case 5
Mrs. Dabrowski Makes Demands and Evokes Guilt

FAMILY MEMBERS AND THEIR PROBLEMS

Mrs. Dabrowski, the identified pateint, is a 70-year-old widow who lives with her son, daughter-in-law, and 15-year-old grandson. The identified patient has a long history of physical difficulties including malabsorption syndrome, diverticulitis, cystitis, arthritis of the neck, Meneires's disease, and possible congestive heart failure. She spent many years caring for her invalid mother and seems to see this as a possible cause of her own difficulties. The nurse noted that Mrs. Dabrowski complains of feeling dizzy and fatigued after visits from friends. Recently she told the nurse that only she understands her and that the doctor never really listens to her.

REASON FOR CONSULTATION

The community health nurse requested that the consultant visit the home with her to determine whether the daughter-in-law thinks that the patient is too demanding. The nurse also expressed concern that the client may have some difficulty that is being overlooked because she is so accustomed to the incessant complaints that Mrs. Dabrowski makes. Lastly, the nurse questioned whether the family had strong feelings toward the nurse because, on her last visit, the daughter-in-law and mother joined forces to attack her. The nurse recalled being anxious when she was attacked by the family and became even more so when she tried to defend her care and the family responded by attacking her more. The nurse also noticed that on several occasions the family became upset when the nurse refused its offer of tea or cake.

The community health nurse had already prepared family members by telling them another nurse would visit with her to observe. The consultant agreed to observe while the community health nurse proceeded with her nursing care.

THE HOME VISIT

During the visit both the elder and younger Mrs. Dabrowski were cordial. Mrs. Dabrowski complained frequently at the beginning of the visit. While doing so, she lowered her head and seemed uncomfortable. When the community health nurse drew up a chair to listen, Mrs. Dabrowski became more animated and told of her discomfort, but also enthusiastically discussed cooking.

The daughter-in-law entered and left the bedroom at intervals, said very little, and played an obedient role in relation to her mother-in-law. Afterward, the consultant and nurse had cake and orange juice in the kitchen with the daughter-in-law. She spoke indirectly of her frustration and possible anger over her mother-in-law's demands.

PROBLEMS IDENTIFIED THROUGH CONSULTATION

The consultant and community health nurse had a long discussion about the family dynamics that seemed to be in operation. One way to view the identified patient's complaining is as a dependency need. She may never have had her own dependency needs met because she had to care for her own mother at an early age. Thus, caring for others and playing the sick role have been a way of life for this woman for many years. It is unlikely that she will give it up readily. The family's cultural expectations about caring for elderly members may also help to maintain Mrs. Dabrowski's complaining behavior and preoccupation with illness.

Rejection seems to play a large part in the dynamics of this family. Family members seem upset when the nurse rejects their offer of tea or cake. They may view the nurse's rejection of food as a rejection of them. Mrs. Dabrowski's constant demands for attention could be a way of proving to herself that she is not rejected, that someone cares.

A final problem area that the nurse related was the constant tendency of the family to cancel appointments, to not want to be disturbed early in the morning, and of Mrs. Dabrowski to tell the nurse to come back later after she had agreed to an appointment time.

Problem	Intervention
1 Orientation to purpose of the visit.	1 Establish the limits of the nurse-family relationship.
	a Collaborate with family members to determine which of the days and times the nurse is free to visit are acceptable to them.
	b When they try to change an agreed-upon time, initiate a discussion to determine why they want to do so.
	c Learn the family's cultural norms and try not to disrupt behaviors unless they are potentially destructive, e.g., accept tea and cake when offered as a way of establishing a relationship with the family.
	d The nurse should examine her own feelings about being attacked by the family and whether the nurse's expectations for the relationship are realistic.
2 Family communication.	2 Spend time listening before attempting to provide logical explanations or to teach. Provide support for the daughter-in-law to verbalize her frustration so that she will be better able to cope with her mother-in-law.
3 Client dependency.	3 Increase the client's independence.
	a Allow the client some time to discuss her physical complaints and some time to discuss cooking and other interests; negotiate with the client in order to determine how this time will be structured.

> b Encourage the client to talk about cooking and her other interests by smiling, nodding, answering in the affirmative, and making positive comments.
> c Design a behavioral contract with the family to encourage the client to cook or plan meals.

EVALUATION

Three weeks after the consultation, the community health nurse wrote the following evaluation:

> Mrs. Dabrowski still makes a lot of demands, but I am less susceptible to them and I feel less threatened when the family gets angry with me; I see this as its way of coping with the situation. It was reassuring for me to get the consultant's confirmation of the family dynamics that I suspected were in operation.

Case 6

Mr. Jones Has Anxiety Attacks

FAMILY MEMBERS AND THEIR PROBLEMS

Mr. Jones, age 66, lives alone next door to his daughter and her family. For 5 years he has devoted himself to caring for his wife. She has had four cerebral vascular accidents and was recently placed in a nursing home by his daughter when Mr. Jones fainted after a hyperventilation episode. His daughter has been telling him for years that the care of his wife is too much for him. About 2 weeks prior to the hyperventilation incident, Mr. Jones fell off a ladder while trying to remove storm windows; there were no apparent injuries. Mrs. Snyder, his daughter, told the community health nurse that "he overdoes it around the house ever since the union forced him to retire." When Mr. Jones retired, he built a house "for my wife" next door to their daughter, but far from their friends and his old work companions. Mrs. Snyder told the nurse that she has had a depressive episode recently because she cannot handle her teenage daughter and the pressure of her parents' health problems at the same time.

REASON FOR CONSULTATION

The community health nurse described feeling helpless and conflicted in regard to this family system. She requested a joint visit where the consultant, nurse, client, and his daughter would meet to discuss the health care issues in the family.

THE HOME VISIT

During the visit, Mr. Jones began breathing very fast whenever his wife was mentioned. Mrs. Synder tried to get the nurses to side with her and to make decisions for her about how to deal with her father, mother, and daughter. During the visit it was agreed that Mrs. Snyder would call a family meeting of her brothers and sisters and their families in order to discuss the pros and cons of keeping Mrs. Jones in the nursing home. Mrs. Snyder seemed relieved that she could share this responsibility with others. Mr. Jones agreed to meet weekly with the mental health nursing specialist to talk about his fainting spells and his relationship with his wife.

PROBLEMS AND INTERVENTIONS IDENTIFIED
THROUGH CONSULTATION

The consultant and community health nurse agreed that the mental health nursing specialist would work with Mr. Jones on the following problems:

Problems	Interventions

1 Client anxiety.	1 Decrease the client's anxiety.
	   a Explore the sources of his anxiety.
	   b Teach him relaxation exercises.

2 Family guilt.	2 Encourage exploration of pros and cons of leaving Mrs. Jones in the nursing home.

3 Client communication.	3 Improve the client's communication skills.
	   a Teach him how to describe his thoughts and feelings.
	   b Help him to use role playing in order to practice verbal communication with others.

EVALUATION

The mental health nursing specialist worked with Mr. Jones once a week for 6 months on an hourly basis. At the end of that time, Mr. Jones no longer had episodes of hyperventilation, was able to accept the idea that he could no longer care for his wife in his home, and had substituted senior citizens' activities for the time he had previously spent caring for his wife.

Case 7
Mrs. Dorsey Has Multiple Sclerosis

FAMILY MEMBERS AND THEIR PROBLEMS

Mrs. Dorsey, the identified patient, was diagnosed as having multiple sclerosis 3 years ago. Her husband contributes to the household by providing money, but is rarely home since his wife became ill. Mrs. Dorsey's 8-year-old son, Tad, is kept home from school by his mother to assist with her morning care. Volunteer workers from her church have organized themselves to offer to care for Mrs. Dorsey so that Tad can go to school on time. Mrs. Dorsey has an 18-year-old daughter who left home because of her mother's demands.

REASON FOR CONSULTATION

Mrs. Dorsey is turning off everybody by her demanding, dependent behavior. The church volunteers want to help, but seem frightened and angry. The community health nurses involved with the family are interested in examining their reactions and in reevaluating their nursing approaches.

GROUP CONSULTATION DISCUSSION

There was a discussion of the two devices that multiple sclerosis patients usually use to compensate for their loss of bodily function. One compensatory device is to become overly independent; the other is to become more demanding and more dependent. Mrs. Dorsey seems to fall into the latter category of m. s. patients. By demanding continual physical supervision, she is able to control her feelings (that are probably overwhelming her) of fear of being abandoned. She is also able to focus on her physical care and to protect herself from experiencing the loss that she has and will incur. Her fear of being abandoned has realistic components. Her daughter has abandoned her, and although her husband remains tied to her financially, he seems physically and emotionally to have separated from her. Lastly, due her lack of mobility, she is quite helpless and dependent on others; this would cause her to be extremely sensitive to any rejection of her or threat to her care.

The nurses identified Mrs. Dorsey's conflict and the signs of it. At one moment she agrees to wait until the nurse arrives, and then changes her mind and demands immediate care. In an effort to deal with her difficulties, she converts her anxiety into anger and belittles all helping efforts. Although Mrs. Dorsey herself focuses only on her physical care, she has remarked several times that others are only concerned about her body, and that "no one understands me." Perhaps because she feels misunderstood, she attempts to play one nurse off against another by telling one how "Mrs. Todd always lets me do it this way" and then telling Mrs. Todd how well the other nurses take care of her.

Mrs. Dorsey's pattern of interaction seems to be to drive others away and then to feel abandoned. She has succeeded in getting her husband, daughter, the physical therapist, and now the nurses and church volunteers to leave her or to at least question their ability to deal with her. This could set up a pattern of mutual withdrawal.

PROBLEMS AND INTERVENTIONS IDENTIFIED THROUGH CONSULTATION

As a result of the group discussion, the following problems and interventions were identified:

Problems	Interventions
1 Client dependency.	1 Increase the client's independence through consistent planning and follow-through. All caregivers will meet to decide on which of Mrs. Dorsey's demands they will be able to meet and will then set limits accordingly.
2 Family interaction.	2 Evaluate, and if necessary, introduce new system boundaries. a Make an appointment to talk with Mr. Dorsey about his view of the situation. b Evaluate Danny's (the son's) reaction to his mother's demands through consultation with the school nurse and/or with Danny.

    c Evaluate and if necessary support or introduce new people for Danny to relate to as sources of parenting and support.

3 Client communication.

3 Begin to focus on Mrs. Dorsey as a person.

    a Pick up on the opening statements that she has made, e.g., "No one understands me," and help to explore the origin of that idea and how the nurse could understand her better.

    b Evaluate the potential for using a Friendly Visitor volunteer who could develop a supportive relationship with Mrs. Dorsey.

EVALUATION

Three weeks after the consultation, the community health nurse reported that the caregivers involved with the family had met to decide on a consistent approach that all would use. The nurse had been unable to reach Mr. Dorsey by telephone, but planned to send him a letter as a way to indicate support and interest in him. A Friendly Visitor had been found to work with Mrs. Dorsey.

Case 8

Billy Has Cerebral Palsy

FAMILY MEMBERS AND THEIR PROBLEMS

Billy Nichols, age 4, is the identified patient. He lives with his mother and father. Mrs. Nichols seems very skeptical about the usefulness of visits from the community health nurse, and frequently refuses to answer the door. Sometimes she speaks to the nurse through the door, and at other times she pretends that she is not home even though the nurse can see her or Billy through the window. Mr. Nichols is never home when the nurse visits, but has answered the telephone on several occasions. The nurse got the impression that he wanted to please her, but that he, too, was skeptical about what, if any, good the nurse's visits could do.

REASON FOR CONSULTATION

The community health nurse expressed anxiety about relating with this family. She stated that she would like to refer the family to agencies that could be helpful to it, but that the family seemed disinterested. She requested a consultation to discuss possible reasons for her inability to reach this family.

PROBLEMS AND INTERVENTIONS IDENTIFIED
THROUGH CONSULTATION

There was a long discussion between the consultant and the community health nurse about the stresses that this family may be under. A major problem seemed to be the parents' conflict over relating with the nurse. Their conflict may have been precipitated or reinforced by their feelings about having produced a defective child. The conflict is evident in Mrs. Nichols's inconsistent behavior: she answers the door, then refuses to answer the door; she talks to the nurse through the door, then answers the door and lets the nurse in. One of the issues that was clarified was the nurse's assumption that Mrs. Nichols is disinterested in or does not like her. The nurse was able to test her theory of disinterest/dislike on one occasion and found that Mrs. Nichols's behavior is inconsistent and unclear. Although the nurse assumed on her last visit that Mrs. Nichols did not want to see her, when she was questioned Mrs. Nichols revealed that it was not that she did not want to see the nurse, but that she was embarrassed about her house being dirty. This example demonstrates how Mrs. Nichols's behavior can be misread by others.

Mrs. Nichols also gives other indirect messages that could be misread or overlooked. For example, she told the nurse several times that "The doctor is only interested in Billy." One possible interpretation of this comment is that it implies "and no one is interested in me." Although Billy is the identified patient, support directed toward the mother will indirectly affect Billy's care.

During the discussion, it was revealed that Mrs. Nichols's mother is rarely available to support her daughter since she has two jobs. The mother would be the natural source of emotional support for the daughter since she lives upstairs and has verbalized a wish to help. Another source of support for Mrs. Nichols is her husband. Through the discussion, it was learned that the nurse had not investigated what assistance he could be to his wife. As the discussion ended, the following problems were identified and interventions agreed upon:

Problems	Interventions
1 Client anxiety about her relationship with the nurse and the appearance of her house.	1 Telephone prior to visit in order to give Mrs. Nichols some option in deciding when the visit will occur.

2 Client conflict.	2 Support the side of Mrs. Nichols's conflict that tends toward seeing the nurse's visits as helpful to her; e.g., pick up on and explore comments such as, "The doctor is only interested in Billy."
3 Unresolved parental grief.	3 Assist both parents to discuss their thoughts and feelings about having a child like Billy.
4 Family need for coping devices.	4 Check the changes that have occurred in family supports. Assess the need to provide new supports or to reinforce already established sources of support.

EVALUATION

A week after the consultation, the community health nurse reported that Mrs. Nichols seemed more open to talking with the nurse about her feelings about being "strapped with a sick kid." The nurse was still trying to determine other sources of support for Mrs. Nichols, but planned to continue to assist the parents to work through their grief about having produced a defective child.

Case 9

Summer Thomas Is Pregnant

REASON FOR CONSULTATION

While working in a school system, a community health nurse was approached by Summer Thomas, a young black girl of 15. Summer confided to the nurse that she was pregnant and wanted to have an abortion without her parents' knowledge. The nurse spoke with Summer about the abortion and made an appointment to speak with her the following week. In the meantime, the nurse received a note from the principal that he had received an irate call from Summer's parents threatening to sue the nurse for withholding information about their daughter from them. The nurse requested a mental health nursing consultation to decide on an appropriate strategy.

PROBLEMS AND INTERVENTIONS IDENTIFIED
THROUGH CONSULTATION

During the consultation, the community health nurse focused primarily on her fear of being sued and on the ethics of the situation. The consultant pointed out that the community health nurse's anxiety about the situation might be preventing her from examining possible sources of anxiety and anger in the clients. With assistance, the nurse was able to see that the threat from Summer's parents might have been due to a conversion of their anxiety about Summer's predicament into anger at her. Once the community health nurse reduced her own anxiety by venting her feelings of anxiety, it was possible to decide how to deal with the Thomas family. The following problems were identified and interventions agreed upon through consultation:

Problems	Interventions
1 Family anxiety/anger.	1 Suggest that the family meet with the community health nurse. a Allow each member to vent his or her thoughts and feelings. b As the family begins to cool down, focus the discussion on how the family intends to handle the issue of Summer's pregnancy.
2 Family communication.	2 Use the family meeting to accomplish the following. a Open up the issue for discussion. b Determine the sequence of events that lead up to the irate phone call. c Assess family supports. d Teach the family more direct communication methods.

EVALUATION

Since emotions were so high, the pros and cons of alternative solutions could not be adequately discussed in one meeting with the family. After one meeting, Summer's parents seemed less angry and agreed to meet with the nurse and Summer the following week for a further discussion of how to handle the pregnancy.

Case 10

Jeremy Park and the School System

FAMILY MEMBERS AND THEIR PROBLEMS

Jeremy Park, age 12, has been skipping school lately. He has Perthe's disease and must wear a leg brace for several years in order to put his hip joint at rest. When Jeremy does go to school, he frequently unhitches his brace or takes it off completely. He has been in several fights with classmates because they call him "Peg Leg." Jeremy's mother is an unemployed school teacher who checks on Jeremy to make sure that he does his exercises, and hollers at him when he does not do them as well or as frequently as she would like him to. Mr. Park is an unemployed factory worker who lets his wife do most of the talking, but at times blows up at Jeremy and tells him that he is no good. Jeremy has a 19-year-old brother, Michael, who is away at college. Mrs. Park called the community health nurse because she feels guilty and depressed that Jeremy is not progressing. She told the nurse that Jeremy is "too much for me to handle."

REASON FOR CONSULTATION

The community health nurse visited the Park home several times. Each time she found herself telling Jeremy to protect his leg and scolding him when he did not follow through with the doctor's orders. She also reported feeling strong pressure from Mrs. Park to do something immediately to change Jeremy's behavior.

PROBLEMS AND INTERVENTIONS IDENTIFIED
THROUGH CONSULTATION

The consultant helped the community health nurse to see that she had been triangled into the family system, and had sided with the parents. The community health nurse agreed that she did feel more comfortable relating with them than with Jeremy who refused to talk to her except to grunt or give an occasional "yes" or "no" when questioned. It was agreed that the community health nurse would continue to provide support for the parents, while at the same time trying to find a person or group to assist Jeremy to find constructive outlets for his normal growth and developmental attempts at independence. Through consultation, the following problems were identified and interventions agreed upon:

Problems	Interventions

1 Parental conflict over Jeremy's behavior.	1 Decrease parental conflict.
	  a Assist both parents to identify the two pulls that they are experiencing, i.e., their wish to be concerned, growth-promoting parents versus their wish to keep Jeremy dependent and obedient to their desires.
	  b Help the parents to examine the pros and cons of each way of relating to Jeremy.

2 Jeremy's normal growth and developmental need for independence.	2 Assist Jeremy to separate from his parents and to grow.
	  a Encourage Jeremy to act independently in some areas of his life.
	  b Discuss Jeremy's reactions to his brace as a possible healthy expression of his independence and need for peer approval.
	  c Help Jeremy's parents to draw up with their son a behavioral contract in order for him to follow the doctor's orders, to involve Mr. Park in monitoring Jeremy's progress, and to reward both parents for allowing their son to be independent.
	  d Find a male role model for Jeremy who can support his attempts at independence.

3 Jeremy's grief over the loss of his body function.	3 Locate a group of 12-year-olds with similar problems for Jeremy to join.

EVALUATION

Three weeks after the initial conference, the community health nurse and consultant met to evaluate the progress that this family had made. The consultant had found a group of 12- to 15-year-olds at a mental health clinic that would accept Jeremy as a member. Jeremy had agreed to go to a group meeting "even though it won't help." Jeremy's brother, Michael, was home for the holidays and the focus of parental concern had shifted to him. The community health nurse had helped the family to draw up a behavioral contract that was agreeable to everyone. The nurse planned to visit with the parents once a month for the next few months and to reevaluate the need for further visits at that time. Although no male role model was found for Jeremy, he seemed to be faring better as evidenced by his missing fewer school days.

Case 11
Mrs. Kettsell Can't Breathe

FAMILY MEMBERS AND THEIR PROBLEMS

Mrs. Kettsell, age 38, has myasthenia gravis. She is in a wheelchair. Her husband expresses concern about her care and recently called the community health nurse for assistance. Mr. Kettsell has a highly responsible job and is rarely home. The Kettsells have two children: Jon, age 16, and Jean, age 15.

REASON FOR CONSULTATION

The community health nurse asked the mental health nursing consultant to make a home visit with her to help determine why the nurse felt so helpless with this family, to determine how much of an emotional component there might be to Mrs. Kettsell's respiratory crises, and to suggest ways in which the community health nurse might communicate more effectively with the client.

THE HOME VISIT

During the home visit, the client's nonverbal communication (expressed through her tone of voice, facial expression, and body language) was inconsistent with her verbal communication, which indicated that she was calm and that all was going well with the family. Her nonverbal communication signaled demands to be helped, taken care of, and sympathized with. A family coping mechanism of denial seemed to be operating both in the client and in other family members. Considering the stress that Mrs. Kettsell is under, such a response is probably to be expected to some degree. Although she verbally denies any need for assistance, her nonverbal messages may be giving a more realistic view of her needs than her verbal ones. Because of this inconsistency in Mrs. Kettsell's verbal and nonverbal messages about her well-being, there is a definite possibility that her respiratory crises may have an emotional component.

This component may reinforce and increase other stressors for Mrs. Kettsell. As her myasthenic symptoms increase, her levels of anxiety and helplessness increase; since she communicates unclearly about her emotional needs, this probably causes additional stress. During the visit, Mrs. Kettsell revealed an added stressor; the recent loss of a supportive friend. Members of Mrs. Kettsell's family probably unknowingly add stress to the system as a result of Mrs. Kettsell's communication with them. They probably feel frustrated and helpless because they are unsure of how Mrs. Kettsell really feels.

Mrs. Kettsell and the nurse may also be giving inconsistent, contradictory messages to each other. Since the family communication system is already unclear, it is imperative that the nurse be clear in her communication.

Another major dynamic operating in the family system and reinforced by the nurse is the element of helplessness. Since helplessness is a feeling that is often contagious, the nurse and other family members may have recognized it and responded to it with their own feelings of helplessness. It is not unusual for people to feel helpless when faced with death and dying; the client has a progressively deteriorating illness process that may be especially difficult for her to accept since she is young and still responsible for the rearing of her children.

PROBLEMS AND INTERVENTIONS IDENTIFIED
THROUGH CONSULTATION

Based on the preconference and home visit, the consultant and community health nurse identified the following problems and agreed upon the following interventions:

Problems	Interventions
1 Client communication.	1 Teach the client how to communicate clearly and effectively. a Provide a role model of clear communication. b Help Mrs. Kettsell to describe and explore her thoughts and feelings. c Clarify confusing or contradictory statements, e.g., say to the client, "You're saying things are OK, but you sound sad."

d Use the process recording
method to pinpoint areas
where the nurse can be more
effective in assisting Mrs.
Kettsell to communicate.

2 Unresolved grief of client.

2 Assist the client to work through
her grief by discussing the effect
on her of recent changes, e.g.,
the loss of her friend, the reaction of family members to her,
her feelings about the illness
process.

EVALUATION

The consultant and community health nurse met the following week to discuss a process recording made by the nurse. Communication between the nurse and client had already become clearer. The nurse stated that she planned to help the client work through her grief in upcoming visits.

Case 12
Mr. Bergman Has a Mid-Career Crisis

FAMILY MEMBERS AND THEIR PROBLEMS

Mrs. Bergman, age 38, was injured in a fall 10 years ago, and is paralyzed below the waist. She has household help, but is able to coordinate the work from her wheelchair. Mr. Bergman is a health research scientist. When he earned his Ph.D. 12 years ago, he was told that he showed great promise as a researcher. Since then he has been unable to complete any original research. Recently he started to romance the wife of one of his colleagues. When the community health nurse visited the Bergman home to change Mrs. Bergman's foley catheter, she asked the nurse to talk with her husband because she was "afraid something is happening to him."

REASON FOR CONSULTATION

The community health nurse asked for a consultation in order to discuss how to approach Mr. Bergman and to speculate on what his behavior might mean.

PROBLEMS AND INTERVENTIONS IDENTIFIED
THROUGH CONSULTATION

The consultant pointed out that it is not unusual for people between the ages of 30 and 40 to question their life goals and whether they have been met. At this time, many people reorient themselves or change their (often) idealistic life goals. Others try to work through this disturbing period by proving themselves in athletic or sexual areas. At the end of the discussion, the community health nurse and the consultant agreed on the following problems and interventions:

Problems	Interventions
1 Unresolved grief of Mr. Bergman.	1 Encourage Mr. Bergman to discuss how his wife's physical condition has affected their relationship. a Pick up and explore any comment related to the client's grief or loss by making a statement such as, "Tell me more about that." b Maintain eye contact with the client during discussions of his grief. In this way, you will show your interest and demonstrate the acceptability of such discussions. c Allow the client to break silences and/or encourage him to go on with the topic. d If the client does not bring up the topic, introduce it by saying something like, "I think it is important for us to talk about how things have changed since your wife's accident."
2 Mr. Bergman's mid-career crisis.	2 Assist the client to discuss what his job expectations were and which of these expectations have been met, and to examine alternative expectations and actions that may result in greater satisfaction for him. Some possible statements to use in this regard are:

a "Tell me a little about you and your work; how has it been going?"

b "When you chose to be a scientist, what were your expectations?" "Have they been fulfilled?"

c "What would help you to be more satisfied with your work?"

d "What prevents (assists) you from being more satisfied?" "How have you dealt with this?" "How else could you deal with it?"

EVALUATION

Following the visit to the Bergman home, the community health nurse stated that although he had initiated the conversation about Mr. Bergman's work, he found it difficult to keep the conversation focused on the topic. The consultant suggested that the nurse complete a process recording of the next visit that they could discuss and use to decide on further goals and interventions.

Case 13

Alvira Adams Bears a Child
Who Fails to Thrive

FAMILY MEMBERS AND THEIR PROBLEMS

Alvira Adams, age 19, lives with her husband, Tom, and their infant daughter, Sophie. Sophie has not been gaining weight, and the pediatrician has expressed concern to the mother. Alvira told the nurse that "He's only interested in Sophie. He treats us like guinea pigs." Alvira called the community health nursing agency to request help with Sophie. Alvira works from 6 to 10 p.m.; during that time, Tom takes care of Sophie. Tom works during the day and has a part-time job on weekends. During the nurse's first visit, Alvira told the nurse that she had no one to talk to and that she was worried that something might happen to Sophie. At the same time, Alvira said, "I don't know what you can do to help" and questioned why the nurse wanted to visit again.

REASON FOR CONSULTATION

The community health nurse expressed concern that Alvira might be an abusive parent, or at least have a high potential for being one. She requested help in evaluating the potential for abusive behavior in this family and in providing appropriate nursing interventions.

PROBLEMS AND INTERVENTIONS IDENTIFIED
THROUGH CONSULTATION

The following problems were discussed and interventions agreed upon:

Problems	Interventions
1 Client conflict over relating with the nurse.	1 Support behaviors that indicate Alvira's interest in working with the nurse, e.g., make statements such as, "I will help you with your concern" and "You said you have no one to talk with; perhaps I can be that person for a while."
2 Client need for coping devices.	2 Evaluate Alvira's potential for child abuse. a Take down a history of Alvira's sources of interpersonal support, of her own family's experiences with abuse, and of how she handles her frustration and anger. b Explore Alvira's fears that something might happen to Sophie. What does she think might happen? Where did she get the idea that something might happen? Has something happened already? c Provide support for Alvira as a way to decrease her potential for abusing Sophie.

d Meet with Alvira and her husband to discuss ways to
improve their communication.
Statements to use to facilitate
this goal include: "Infants
can be frustrating." "It sometimes helps to talk about
your frustration."

e Find referral sources for
Alvira and her family such
as self-help programs and/or
counseling services.

EVALUATION

A week after the consultation, the community health nurse wrote that, although
Alvira still seemed overly anxious about her child, she had agreed to go with
Tom for counseling at the mental health clinic.

Case 14

Henry Is a Quadriplegic

FAMILY MEMBERS AND THEIR PROBLEMS

Mr. Isone is a 26-year-old man who became quadriplegic as the result of an
accident 10 years ago. He worked as an insurance agent until last summer
when he developed chronic skin and elimination problems. The community
health nurses and Mr. Isone's mother refer to him as "Henry," although it is
not clear that he prefers to be addressed in this manner. Mr. Isone is described
as very involved with his mother by the nurses. Mrs. Isone takes care of all his
physical needs (including turning him every 2 hours) and both mother and
son spend a great deal of time talking about food and elimination.

When Mr. Isone's sister-in-law had her baby, the client stopped putting
out urine and was planning to go into the hospital. When his mother demonstrated to him that she was still able to care for him, he resumed his urine
output. Now Mr. Isone's aunt is planning to move nearby; the nurse wonders
whether this move might be a possible threat to the relationship of Mr. Isone
and his mother.

Both Mr. Isone and the community health nurse express concern over (but
not to) Mrs. Isone. She has hypertension and no outside diversions to provide

her with support. The client's father works nights and sleeps days; he is not involved in Mr. Isone's care. The nurse has noticed that the father has temper tantrums and throws household objects when he becomes angry.

The nurses characterize the identified patient as socially inept and describes him as wanting interpersonal contact, but shying away from it. He frequently calls friends or the nurse and makes a date or appointment, and then cancels it. His communication skills primarily include asking the nurse questions about herself.

REASON FOR CONSULTATION

Several community health nurses requested a group consultation to share information and to decide on a consistent series of interventions for this family. They expressed helplessness and confusion about relating to the Isone family.

PROBLEMS AND INTERVENTIONS IDENTIFIED
THROUGH CONSULTATION

During the group consultation it became clear that the community health nurses were reflecting some of the feelings and reactions of the Isone family. For example, their feelings of helplessness and conflict were reactions that Mr. Isone demonstrated through his physical inability to care for himself and through his pattern of approaching and avoiding interpersonal contacts by setting up appointments and then canceling them.

Another problem that was identified through consultation was the infantilization of Mr. Isone by those around him and how the way in which the nurses were addressing him may reinforce his tendency toward taking on a life-long sick role of dependency.

Another major problem seemed to be the rigid relationships among family members, and their attempt at this point to triangle in the nurse. There was a discussion about why the family may be requesting additional help at this time. It was speculated that Mr. Isone may be increasingly anxious about the possible loss of his relationship with his mother and also angry that his physical predicament and lack of social skills prevent him from establishing extrafamily relationships.

As a result of the discussion, the following problems were identified and interventions agreed upon:

Problems	Interventions
1 Orientation to purpose of the visit.	1 Set limits on the nurse-client relationship and follow through on agreed-upon goals.
	a Determine by what name Mr. Isone prefers to be addressed

and then address him by that name.

    b Ask family how nurse can be helpful now and why the family has requested help at this time.

2 Mr. Isone's conflict.

2 Examine parts of the client's conflict and support his constructive behaviors.

    a Assist the client to discuss the two pulls that he is experiencing.

    b Reward the client when he follows through on an agreed-upon appointment.

3 Client need for coping devices.

3 Strengthen the client's social skills and teach him new ones.

    a Reward constructive interpersonal attempts on the part of the client.

    b Set up role playing and/or structured communication exercises to teach him social skills.

    c Teach the client to resume more of his own physical care.

    d Determine what other family members or friends could get involved in Mr. Isone's physical care.

4 Client anxiety.

4 Evaluate the sources of the client's anxiety and teach him ways to decrease it.

    a Explore the sources of his anxiety, especially in relation to his mother.

    b Teach him relaxation exercises and how to problem-solve.

5 Family interaction.

5 Promote the separateness of family members.

    a Support extrafamily interactions for Mrs. Isone and her son.

        b Develop a relationship with Mrs. Isone as a way to allow her to separate from her son.

        c Plan extrafamily events that lead to the separateness of family members.

        d Talk with the father alone, encouraging him to verbalize his thoughts and feelings as a way to decrease his need to act these out by throwing objects.

EVALUATION

In a follow-up discussion, the community health nurses revealed that they had determined that the client preferred to be called Mr. Isone and that he was pleased that he had been consulted about this. The nurses had begun to develop role-playing and communication exercises to assist the client to develop his social skills. The nurses had convinced Mrs. Isone to purchase a water bed so that her son would need to be turned less often. Mrs. Isone had become more involved with her sister-in-law, and her son had begun to form a relationship with a young man with multiple sclerosis who represented the Overcomers, a self-help group for handicapped people. The nurses reported that they had been unsuccessful in talking with the client's father who stated that he was too tired to talk in the daytime because he worked all night. The nurses expressed fewer feelings of helplessness and conflict, and were now goal-directed.

Case 15

Mrs. Florio Is Intimidating

FAMILY MEMBERS AND THEIR PROBLEMS

Mr. Florio has had several cerebral vascular accidents. The doctor has called him hopeless. The community health nurse has observed that his wife treats him like an object; she cares for his physical needs, but does not talk with him when the nurse is there. The sicker Mr. Florio is, the more upset his wife gets and the more demands she makes on the nurses. She blames them for being late or for not providing adequate care for her husband.

REASON FOR CONSULTATION

Several nurses work with the Florios. All have had strong emotional reactions to working with them. Some seem angry about the demands that the family makes and are especially upset that the family does not seem to appreciate the care that it has received. Others are intimiated by Mrs. Florio's anger and express feelings of helplessness and hopelessness about the situation. They view the family as unhealthy and hopeless.

PROBLEMS AND INTERVENTIONS IDENTIFIED THROUGH CONSULTATION

Emotions were high during the group consultation. It was agreed that Mrs. Florio is converting her anxiety about the possible loss of her husband, and her guilt that his debility may be her fault, into anger, and is displacing or projecting that anger on to the nurses. Once the source of intimidation was identified, the nurses seemed more able to focus on family strengths and on potential ways to intervene with this family. For example, it was noted that Mrs. Florio had taken several constructive steps including planning and implementing a spring vacation for her and her husband. Once the nurses were able to identify a family strength, they were more able to place intimidating and seemingly hopeless communications in perspective.

The problems and interventions that were identified through consultation were:

Problems	Interventions
1 Nurses' reactions to the family system.	1 The nurses must examine their own reactions to anger and helplessness. They can ask themselves the following questions: a Is it necessary to feel hopeless because the doctor and family do? b What is so intimidating about anger? c Why does the nurse need to be thanked for providing a paid service? d Can the nurses begin to listen to Mrs. Florio's words rather than tuning into her affect?

2 Mrs. Florio's anxiety.

2 Decrease client anxiety.
   a Sit down to talk with Mrs. Florio.
   b Refocus the conversation when Mrs. Florio makes a fast change of subject.
   c Examine the source of her anxiety, e.g., make a remark such as, "You seem upset; let's talk about it."
   d Tell Mrs. Florio exactly what the nurse plans to do and when she or he plans to do it, and then see to it that the plan is carried out.

EVALUATION

The next week, the nurses reported that although there had been little change in the family system, they felt less hopeless and intimidated. Several commented that being able to identify and share their feelings about clients helps to separate out what difficulties are due to the nurses' reactions to the family, and what difficulties are due to the family's needs.

Part Four

Case Studies
for Practice

Practice Case 1
Which of Mrs. Gottiglioni's Needs Should Take Priority?

Mrs. Gottiglioni is a 72-year-old woman who has had multiple cerebral vascular accidents. Her left side is paralyzed. For the past year she has been unable to stand or to speak. She moves from bed to wheelchair via lift. Mr. Gottiglioni has recently shared his feelings about his wife with the community health nurse, and has asked for assistance in decreasing his wife's wailing behavior. She wails the loudest when she is placed in unpredictable situations. One community health nurse suggested the use of behavioral modification to decrease Mrs. Gottiglioni's wailing, but thinks that bladder training should be tried first. The nurse also questions whether there may be so much organic brain damage that Mrs. Gottiglioni may be unable to understand directions.

Mr. Gottiglioni has noticed that his wife has two cries; one is high-pitched, which he calls her "fear cry" and the other is lower in register, which he refers to as her "attention-getting cry." Although the client is beginning to verbalize more frequently, her husband continues to try to anticipate and interpret her needs without encouraging her to articulate them.

STUDY QUESTIONS

1 How can the community health nurse test the degree of Mrs. Gottiglioni's organic brain damage?
2 What tests or questions could be used to encourage Mrs. Gottiglioni to practice relating interpersonally?
3 How can the nurse verify Mr. Gottiglioni's hunch that his wife has two types of cries?
4 How can the nurse decide whether bladder training or behavior modification to decrease Mrs. Gottiglioni's wailing should take precedence in her care plan?
5 What healthy behaviors or strengths does this family have?
6 What effects on the family system might Mrs. Gottiglioni's increasing verbalizations of her needs have?
7 What verbal communications can the nurse use to decrease the client's wailing behavior?
8 What information could the nurse give Mr. Gottiglioni to help him to increase his wife's independence?
9 What information does the nurse need about Mr. Gottiglioni's reaction to his wife's crying?
10 What specific statements would you use to gather this information?
11 What information about this case should be shared among health caregivers?
12 What would be the effect of ignoring Mrs. Gottiglioni's cries?

13 What behavioral modification program would you establish in order to decrease Mrs. Gottiglioni's crying?
14 If you were working with this family, would you support the separateness or closeness of family members, or both? What interventions would you make?

Practice Case 2

Antonia Vasquez Is Dying

Antonia Vasquez is 48 years old and single. She has inoperable cancer of the uterus. She has refused cobalt therapy on the grounds that she has had several relatives who had this treatment and who, as a result, had been incontinent, nauseated, and unable to hold their food down. Antonia lives with her father who has severely restricted vision. The community health nurse has known the family for 7 years. Seven years ago, the nurse saw Antonia's stepmother in the emergency room after she had fallen due to an exacerbation of her condition of rheumatoid arthritis. A cervical vertebra collapsed at the time of the fall, and the stepmother became quadraplegic. Antonia took complete care of her step-mother for several years until she developed vasculitis and died in the hospital.

Antonia's father has taken the nurse aside to complain that he cannot deal with the bouts of pain that Antonia has. Dilaudid has no effect on her pain. According to her father, when Antonia is in pain, it is as though she is possessed by demons. At that time, she curses at her father and tells him that she hopes he rots in hell.

The community health nurse has noticed that Antonia's father either hovers over her or else ignores her. When Antonia asks for a tub bath, he refuses, claiming that she is too weak. The nurse states, "I think her father is interfering with Antonia, but I don't know how to stop it." At the same time, the nurse echoes the father's puzzlement over how to be helpful to Antonia.

STUDY QUESTIONS

1 At what stage in the grief process is Antonia?
2 At what stage in the grief process is her father?
3 How can you explain Antonia's anger with her father?
4 What other unresolved griefs and losses might Antonia have?
5 Would you support the current relationship between Antonia and her father or would you try to change it? What specific interventions would you use to introduce change?
6 How do you explain the nurse's feelings of helplessness?   What interventions could be made to change these feelings?

7 How would you respond if Antonia's father confided in you that he cannot take Antonia's attacks of pain? What specific communication responses would help you to gather data from him? What specific communication responses would help the father once you had gathered this information?

8 How could you include Antonia and her father in planning treatment goals?

Practice Case 3
Why Doesn't the DeGroos Family Keep Its Appointments?

Mr. and Mrs. DeGroos wandered into the senior citizens' health care station, which was staffed by several community health nurses. They were unsure about why they had come or what they should expect. One nurse took their blood pressures and began to take down their respective health histories. Before the interview had been completed, the DeGrooses said that they had to leave. The community health nurse made an appointment with them to return the following week. The couple did not appear for 2 weeks. The nurse was both concerned and angry about this, but did not investigate the reason behind her clients' failure to keep their appointment.

The next week, Mr. DeGroos appeared at the health care station 5 minutes before closing time. He told the community health nurse that he had come to complete his health history. The nurse told him that the station was about to close but offered to set up another appointment for him for the following week. The next week both clients appeared, but they arrived an hour later than the agreed-upon time, and Mrs. DeGroos didn't seem to want to be there at all. She made comments aside to her husband such as, "This is just like it was in the hospital," "They won't treat us any better here," and "If nurses are so great, how come they let me fall out of bed in the hospital?"

STUDY QUESTIONS

1 How else might the community health nurse have handled the DeGrooses initially, for example, when they were unsure about why they had come to the station or what they should expect? What specific comments could help to orient the DeGrooses and to establish a working relationship between them and the nurse?

2 Assuming that the DeGrooses were in conflict, what might the nurse have said or done when they got up to leave during their first interview?

3 How else might the nurse have acted when the DeGrooses did not appear for their follow-up appointment? (Consider the possible use of written and telephone communication.)

4 How do you explain the nurse's anger? What interventions would be desirable for the nurse to make in order to deal with her own anger?
5 What is your opinion about the way in which the community health nurse dealt with Mr. DeGroos when he appeared 5 minutes before closing time? How else might the nurse have handled the situation?
6 What specific response might the nurse make to each of the following comments by Mrs. DeGroos?
   a "This is just like it was in the hospital."
   b "They won't treat us any better here."
   c "If nurses are so great, how come they let me fall out of bed in the hospital?"
7 How could you include the DeGrooses in planning treatment goals?

Practice Case 4
Why Isn't Mr. Meck Motivated?

Mr. Meck, 37, is recovering from being hospitalized for a myocardial infarct. Before his hospitalization, Mr. Mech was the president of his own company, and worked 15 hours a day. While he was in the hospital, the nurses complained that Mr. Meck would not stay in bed, and that he was constantly trying to work when his physician wanted him to rest.

The community health nurse came in contact with Mr. Meck at the cardiac clinic. He noticed that Mr. Meck frequently canceled his appointments, and that, when he did come to the clinic, he argued with the nurse about nursing procedure and the doctor's orders and constantly tested the nurse to see whether he meant what he said. The nurse reported feeling torn between wanting to help Mr. Meck to become more independent and wanting to follow the physician's orders. After several unsuccessful attempts to convince Mr. Meck to follow his diet, the community health nurse began to think that the client was not motivated to assist in his own health care.

STUDY QUESTIONS

1 How do you explain Mr. Meck's behavior in the hospital?
2 Which of his needs was he attempting to meet?
3 To which of his needs did the hospital nurses give priority?
4 What is the client's role in deciding which of his needs should be met?
5 How would you decide which needs of the client should receive priority?
6 How do you explain Mr. Meck's canceling of his appointments?
7 How can Mr. Meck's arguing with the nurse be explained in terms of his attempting to control their relationship?

8 The testing behavior of Mr. Meck is characteristic of what phase of the nurse-client relationship?

9 Did the community health nurse seem to be aware that Mr. Meck's testing was a behavior that he should have expected? How else would you have handled this phase of the nurse-client interaction?

10 What concept explains the nurse's feeling of being torn between two goals? What nursing interventions would help to resolve this problem?

11 How could communication techniques have been used with Mr. Meck? State specific comments that you would have made.

12 How would you devise a behavioral contract between you and Mr. Meck? (Consider specific behavioral modification strategies for reinforcing healthy behaviors.) Draw up such a contract.

Practice Case 5

Andrew Has a Body Image Problem

Andrew is a 6-year-old with nephrotic syndrome. He is taking steroids, and although he is supposedly stabilized on the medication, he continues to gain weight. The kids at school call him "Fatty," and his mother claims that as soon as he gets home from school he starts to eat. The community health nurse says that Andrew's mother's knowledge of nutrition is good but that her application of the principles of nutrition is poor. When Andrew is sick and home from school, he eats even more.

The community health nurse thinks that Andrew's weight problem is not a family one since Andrew's mother is quite thin, and his sister weighs a normal amount. The nurse would like to help Andrew to plan his diet, but questions whether this is an activity that would be too complex for him.

The nurse had Andrew draw himself (human figure drawing test) and had the drawing analyzed by another nurse with expertise in this area. The recommendation was that Andrew should obtain psychiatric counseling.

STUDY QUESTIONS

1 Based on your knowledge of obesity and your knowledge of the side effects of steroids, how do you explain Andrew's continuing weight gain?

2 How do you explain the nurse's characterization of the mother's knowledge of nutrition as good but her application of the principles as poor in terms of the nurse's perception?

3 How could the community health nurse validate her hunch that Andrew's problem is a nutritional one?

4 Why might Andrew have a body image problem?
5 How might the nurse work with Andrew to help solve such a body image problem?
6 Drawing on your knowledge of growth and development, do you think that a 6-year-old is too young to understand the principles of nutrition?
7 How might the community health nurse work with Andrew's family?
8 How might the community health nurse work with the school nurse?
9 How might the community health nurse work with Andrew's teacher?
10 Would you want to work with Andrew at school or in his home? Give a rationale for either answer.

Practice Case 6
Mr. Garnett Drinks

Mrs. Garnett is a 23-year-old wife and mother who came to the well child clinic with her 2-year-old son, Ross, whom she says is "too much for me to handle." When the community health nurse first met Mrs. Garnett, the client revealed that she had had a psychiatric hospitalization at age 18 and was concerned about being a good mother. Mrs. Garnett was not specific about the events surrounding her hospitalization, and the community health nurse did not ask her to elaborate. Mr. Garnett, 35, works long hours as a construction worker. Around the time of Ross's birth, Mr. Garnett began to drink. It is not clear to what degree Mrs. Garnett contributed to her husband's drinking by withdrawing physically and emotionally from him after Ross's birth.

Mrs. Garnett complained to the community health nurse that she does not want to stay with her husband because he hits her, denigrates her, and threatens to commit her to a psychiatric facility whenever he is drunk. Mrs. Garnett revealed that Mr. Garnett's mother frequently gives her son money for liquor or buys him a bottle when he visits her, and then complains when he gets drunk. Although Mrs. Garnett said she wanted to leave, she also said that there was nowhere for her to go, and that her husband is always apologetic after his drinking bouts "so maybe he'll reform."

STUDY QUESTIONS

1 How would you interpret Mrs. Garnett's spontaneous comments about having had a psychiatric hospitalization? What specific facilitative questions could you use to elicit more information about her hospitalization?
2 How do you explain Mr. Garnett's drinking in terms of family systems theory?

3 Analyze the Garnett family in terms of Berne's game theory.
   a Who plays the role of Rescuer?
   b Who plays the role of Patsy?
   c Who plays the role of Persecutor?
   d Who plays the role of Connection?
4 What information about the process of psychiatric commitment might you give to Mrs. Garnett?
5 What information about Mrs. Garnett's parenting ability would you need to gather? How would you phrase your questions in order to make them facilitative?
6 How would you determine the support systems that are available to this family?
7 What are the referral sources that you might consider for this family?

Practice Case 7

Is Mr. Hose Hopeless?

Mr. Hose is 75 and lives in a single-room occupancy hotel. The community health nurse was beginning to establish a health clinic in that hotel. She met Mr. Hose in the hallway one day and invited him to a health discussion group that she was leading that evening. He declined, saying that he did not feel up to being with other people. As they were conversing, another resident passed by and said, "Oh, don't bother with him; he's hopeless!" The next week the community health nurse decided to talk with Mr. Hose to find out what his problem was. The following is a process recording of their conversation.

Client: I'm the most depressed person you ever saw.
Nurse: How's that?
Client: I just don't want to do anything.
Nurse: Sometimes we have to make ourselves do things; it often helps.
Client: Well, I don't know . . .
Nurse: Have you gone out this week?
Client: I've been very defiant.
Nurse: In what way?
Client: (silence)
Nurse: You mean someone here has asked you to do something?
Client: Yes, but I look and feel so awful.
Nurse: Oh, you look all right.
Client: I worry about everything.
Nurse: About what for instance?
Client: Oh, about being mugged by the people here, and that I won't get enough to eat.

PRACTICE EXERCISE

Rephrase the following nurse statements and give a rationale for each.

1 "Sometimes we have to make ourselves do things; it often helps."

   Restatement:

   Rationale:

2 "Have you gone out this week?"

   Restatement:

   Rationale:

3 "You mean someone here has asked you to do something?"

   Restatement:

   Rationale:

4 "Oh, you look all right."

   Restatement:

   Rationale:

Practice Case 8
What Does the Condor Family Want?

Mrs. Condor, 75, lives with her son and daughter-in-law. Mrs. Condor has taken cathartics for the past 20 years. During that time, she has slowly been experiencing increased bowel cramping and decreased muscle tone. She hyperventilates, perspires freely while sitting on the toilet after an enema, and appears to be in a state of severe anxiety. The community health nurse becomes anxious and angry because Mrs. Condor will not follow instructions. Mrs. Condor's doctor is on vacation for a month and her son has called the nurse frequently this past week to ask her to give his mother an enema. When the nurse arrived, the family refused to let her in and suggested that she return in a few days. The client's son has an ulcer that has flared up since he lost his job last week and while he frequently says "yes" to the nurse's suggestions, he rarely follows through on them. His wife contradicts her husband at times, but does not usually involve herself with the nurse.

STUDY QUESTIONS

1 What nursing interventions can you think of that would help to relieve Mrs. Condor's anxiety?
2 How do you explain the nurse's reaction to Mrs. Condor's behavior?
3 What recent changes or losses may be affecting this family system now?
4 What devices are family members using to cope with stress?
5 How can the nurse assess the family's need for additional sources of support at this time?
6 What concept would best explain the family's asking the nurse to come and then not admitting her when she arrived? What nursing intervention is called for?
7 How could the nurse persuade family members to work with her toward agreed-upon goals? How would you introduce this as a topic of discussion for this family?

Practice Case 9
Joni Has VD

Joni is 14 and very physically mature for her age. She has contracted gonorrhea. She was referred to the community health nurse for sex education counseling. At the meeting, Joni flirts with the nurse, telling him that he is cute. The nurse finds Joni very attractive and becomes anxious during the discussion, which features Joni's nonchalant and provocative description of her sexual encounter. The community health nurse notes that Joni is mistaken about some areas of sexual functioning and is ignorant of others. For example, Joni states that she has had intercourse, but is uncertain about how she has contracted VD.

At the end of the first session, the nurse realizes that they have spent little time discussing matters of sex education, and that Joni's need for both information and interpersonal relationships is great. They agree to an appointment for the following day. After reflecting for a while, the community health nurse admits that he is very confused about the process of the interview and needs assistance in identifying what disrupted the nurse-client relationship and prevented the goal of the meeting from being reached.

STUDY QUESTIONS

1 How do you explain the nurse's feeling of anxiety while he was interviewing the client?
2 What kinds of information would you gather if you were interviewing Joni? Formulate specific questions that you would ask her.
3 Given the level of your knowledge of the client and the process of the first interview, how many sessions do you think would be necessary for the community health nurse to plan with her?
4 What specific goals would you have for this client?
5 Discuss incidents where you have been sexually aroused by and/or were physically attracted to a client. What were the circumstances of the incident? How did you deal with the situation?
6 What are the ethical ramifications of becoming sexually involved with a client?
7 What steps can you take to decrease the potential of your acting on any sexual fantasies that you may have about clients?
8 How could mental health consultation assist the community health nurse to deal with this client?

Practice Case 10

Ms. Werner Finds a Lump in Her Breast

Angela Werner is a 27-year-old model who has no family nearby and who recently discovered a lump in her left breast. She called the community health nursing agency and asked for information about a breast examination. When the secretary asked her to come by to pick up the information, Ms. Werner agreed.

The community health nurse found Ms. Werner in the hallway clutching the brochure and crying. She agreed to an interview with the nurse. For the first 15 minutes, the client cried and jumped from topic to topic. Finally, Ms. Werner stopped crying and told the nurse that she had found a lump in her breast. The nurse told her what a biopsy entailed and talked with her about various kinds of breast surgery. The nurse then ended the interview after referring the client to several physicians.

The following week, Ms. Werner called the community health nurse and asked her for information about biopsy and breast surgery. The nurse responded that they had discussed those topics during their last meeting and that if she had any questions to ask her physician.

STUDY QUESTIONS

1 How else might the community health nurse have dealt with finding Ms. Werner crying in the hallway?

2 What concept explains Ms. Werner's crying, her jumping from topic to topic, and her inability to retain information?

3 Why might discovering a lump in her breast be especially upsetting for this client? (Consider the nature of the client's stress and the amount of support available to her.)

4 What kinds of information would you have gathered from Ms. Werner? What specific questions would you have asked her?

5 How else could the community health nurse have handled referring the client to a physician?

6 How might the secretary be trained to answer the requests of callers for information so as to respond to the needs of those who might need nursing care? Formulate a specific plan for teaching the secretary this skill.

Practice Case 11

Geraldine Is an Obese Teenager

Geraldine was referred to the community health nurse by her priest. He was concerned about her obesity and had heard her complain that her being overweight was ruining her social life. The nurse agreed to set up an appointment to see Geraldine at her school.

During the meeting, the community health nurse weighed Geraldine and discovered that she was 100 pounds overweight. Geraldine remarked that she did not know that she weighed so much and claimed that she hardly ate anything at all. The nurse asked Geraldine to keep track of everything that she ate and gave her a notebook in which she could make her entries. The nurse also arranged for Geraldine to weigh herself daily at school since the client had no scale at home. Geraldine agreed to sign a contract with the nurse to lose 5 pounds. The nurse asked Geraldine about her sources of exercise, and found that Geraldine was participating in the physical education program at her school. The nurse also asked Geraldine to make a list of the activities that she enjoyed.

STUDY QUESTIONS

1 In addition to determining Geraldine's food intake, what other information do you think would be important to gather in this case?

2 If you were the community health nurse, what information about Geraldine as a person would you want to gather?
3 How would you assist Geraldine to participate successfully in the following interventions:
   a making it difficult for her to overeat
   b decreasing the number of times per day she eats
   c decreasing the number of areas where she eats
   d making eating time only for eating
   e increasing her energy output
4 What concept best explains Geraldine's comment that she hardly ate anything?
5 How would you set up a baseline data graph for Geraldine?
6 What principles of reinforcement would you use with Geraldine? How would you apply them?
7 Draw up a sample contract between the community health nurse and the client.

Practice Case 12
The Parker Infant Dies

Lisa and Jim Parker had a premature infant that died shortly after it was brought home. The community health nurse was making a routine visit to new parents when she stopped by the Parker home. She found Lisa Parker in her pajamas and robe. Dishes were piled in the sink and clothes were strewn throughout the house. When the nurse asked about the infant, Mrs. Parker burst into tears and started to tell the nurse that she could have saved the infant if only she had been a better mother. The nurse assured her that she had been a good mother. At that point, Mrs. Parker seemed to calm down but then became angry and told the nurse that she didn't need her and to please leave.

As the nurse was leaving, Mr. Parker came home from work. He was very quiet, but polite to the nurse. She asked how he was doing, and he said, "Well, it's hard to describe; I just can't believe it happened." The nurse said that she was leaving now, but would return the following day.

STUDY QUESTIONS

1 At what stage in the grief process is Mrs. Parker?
2 How do you explain Mrs. Parker's statement that she could have saved the infant if only she had been a better mother?
3 What are the pros and cons of the nurse's reassuring the mother? What other responses might the nurse have made to Mrs. Parker?

4 How do you explain Mrs. Parker's anger in terms of both grief and communication theory?
5 How else might the nurse have responded to Mr. Parker's statement?
6 What information does the nurse need to gather about the Parkers' need for household help, their systems of support, their stages of grieving, and how they relate to one another? How would you use facilitative questions to systematically gather this information?
7 How would you include Mr. and Mrs. Parker in formulating treatment goals? What exactly would you say to them to make the relationship a collaborative one?
8 How might you help the Parkers to resolve their grief? What other resources or referral sources might you use?

Practice Case 13

Jake Experiments with Drugs

Jake Olson is 16 years old. He was recently released from the hospital after a bout of serum hepatitis. Both he and his 14-year-old sister are adopted. Jake's mother works full-time and refers to Jake as her "problem child who I can't control." He was arrested for possession of heroin and a stolen gun. He was placed in the children's shelter but escaped. The judge has agreed to place Jake in a residential treatment center if it can be arranged. Mrs. Olson told the community health nurse that she noticed "changes" in Jake since last summer. She attributed these changes to his use of drugs. Mr. Olson has washed his hands of Jake and refuses to discuss him anymore, claiming that his foster son is just bad. In Mrs. Olson's opinion, Jake does these things because he's angry about learning that he was adopted. The community health nurse tried to talk to Jake about what he is doing to himself and to his family, as well as about the dangers of drug abuse, but he would not listen. The community health nurse is angry with the family because they did not listen to her suggestion to place Jake in a residential treatment center earlier. The nurse has set up an appointment with the Olson family to discuss the residential treatment center idea more fully.

STUDY QUESTIONS

1 In terms of family systems theory, what purpose might Jake's behavior serve?
2 Even though you have never met Jake, do you think less of him because he uses heroin rather than Valium or beer?

3 Using Huberty's theory of drug abusing families (Chapter 7) what assessments and interventions would you plan in the following areas?
   a tendency to deny drug effects
   b ignorance of the effects of drug use
   c failure to accept responsibility
   d inability to communicate thoughts and feelings
   e parental drug abuse
4 If you were able to work with this family, how would you enlist their collaboration?
5 How could you help Jake to resolve his feelings about being adopted? What are some of the problems involved?

Practice Case 14

Merritt Is Hyperactive

Merritt is an 8-year-old whom his teacher has labelled "hyperactive." Merritt is an only child who does not relate to his peers except for a girl in his class with whom he fights and argues. His parents are well educated, and stress intellectual skills. They feel uncomfortable hugging Merritt and talking with him except to reward him for good grades. His mother says that she is "overwhelmed" by her son and cannot handle it when he runs around or plays roughly.

The community health nurse became involved with Merritt when his teacher asked for assistance. The teacher said that Merritt is set apart from the others in the classroom because of his religion. He is a Jehovah's Witness and is not allowed to join in when the Pledge of Allegiance is said or to attend the birthday parties of his classmates. The teacher also related her feeling that she can't control Merritt in class. When the community health nurse and the teacher began to work together, they agreed to try social learning methods with Merritt in school, but then the teacher changed her mind and claimed that such a technique was cruel. The nurse observed the teacher in the classroom and noted that she did use punishment and reward, but did so inconsistently.

The nurse also met with the teacher and Merritt's mother, but the teacher contradicted everything that the nurse said. The nurse became very angry and decided to work only with Merritt and his mother.

STUDY QUESTIONS

1 How might the community health nurse help determine whether Merritt is hyperactive? Research the definition of hyperactivity and make a study of the controversy surrounding this term.

2 What further information might you need to gather about Merritt's behavior in the classroom?
3 How might you work with the teacher to decrease her feelings of conflict?
4 How might you work with the teacher to teach her how to apply social learning methods to the entire class so that Merritt would not be singled out?
5 What further information would you need to gather from Merritt and his family?
6 What might Merritt's parents need to know about growth and development and parenting skills?

Practice Case 15

Susan Is Anxious About School

Susan is a six-year-old who comes to the nurse's office frequently with various physical complaints. Most often she complains of stomach pains of unknown origin. Susan's mother has taken her to several doctors, but they all think that the problem is psychological.

When the community health nurse talked with Susan's teacher, she was told that Susan was opinionated and dogmatic. The teacher told the nurse that Susan was unable to tolerate others' ideas or play. The teacher noted that Susan related most easily with adults, and was likely to try to charm them by presenting sophisticated ideas or to shock them by telling stories of how her father was shot in the head and killed. Evidently, Susan's mother had remarried and her stepfather had adopted her, but Susan acted as if she had no father.

When the nurse spoke with Susan's mother, she confirmed what the teacher had said. She added that Susan had begun to have physical complaints at the time of her father's death. The nurse made no attempt to investigate what the mother had told Susan about the circumstances of her father's death. Susan's mother told the nurse that at times she felt as if she was the child when Susan called her grandmother to report that "Mommy has been bad."

STUDY QUESTIONS

1 How do you explain Susan's physical complaints if there is no organic basis for them? What nursing intervention might be useful?
2 How else might the nurse have handled Susan's coming to her office complaining of pain?
3 What further information does the nurse need to gather about Susan's behavior with peers? What interventions would you suggest as a way to help Susan to develop cooperative play with others?

4 What would be the most useful way to respond to Susan's shocking stories or sophisticated ideas?
5 What sources of unresolved grief might Susan have? What nursing interventions would you suggest?
6 How could the nurse work with Susan and her family? (Consider the use of role reversal, how change could be introduced, and what interventions the nurse might make.)

Part Five

Simulated Situations
for Practice

Simulation 1
My Favorite Family Roles

This simulation requires seven or eight players. Each player chooses a role closest to the one that he or she plays in his or her own family. There may be some roles that are more popular than others; bargain with other group members for the role that you want to play, or, if your favorite role has been taken, start another group where you can play that role.

When the players have read the part descriptions below, they are to choose their roles, and then decide on and plan a family activity together. The roles available are:

Player A You are always getting into trouble. You don't think that you behave that differently from other family members, but somehow everyone picks out your flaws, or defines your behavior as bad or unacceptable. Whenever anything goes wrong in the family, you get blamed for it.

Player B You use humor to defuse emotional situations. You clown around a lot and are never serious. Whenever a disagreement starts, you tell a joke, tease people for being too serious, or act in a humorous fashion.

Player C You are always trying to do things for others. Whenever anyone indicates either by word or by gesture that he or she is about to attempt a task or to make a decision, you jump in to take charge and try to do it for him or her.

Player D You make sure that others understand one another. You relay comments between people whenever there is indirect communication. You try to clarify messages by telling one person what the other person meant.

Player E You choose one of the other players and agree with whatever he says, side with him against all the others, and try to form a mutually exclusive relationship with that person.

Player F You go around telling people what they should do and how they should think and feel. You are not concerned with their ideas and when they start to tell you their thoughts or feelings, you immediately tell them your ideas on the subject.

Player G Whenever a disagreement begins, you rush in to make peace. You are very uncomfortable with the expression of anger, and want to change the mood to one of conciliation as soon as possible. Although you might not say so, you often wonder if you are not the cause of many disagreements.

Player H You are the timekeeper. You begin the simulation when all the other players have signalled you that they are ready to begin. You start the simulation and keep it going for 15 minutes. After 15 minutes, you call "Time," and then lead the group discussion using the following questions.

DISCUSSION QUESTIONS

1 Assessments
  a Who played the problem child role?
  b Who played the joker role?
  c Who played the messenger role?
  d Who played the advice-giver role?
  e Who played the peacemaker role?
  f Who played the helper role?
  g Who played the ally role?
  h What triangles developed?
  i What myths did this family have?
  j Which relationships were symmetrical?
  k Which relationships were complementary?
  l What behaviors of others helped you to maintain you role?
  m What behaviors of others prevented you from maintaining your role?
  n Who detracted from completing the assigned task? How?
2 Interventions
  a How could you change your assigned role so as to accomplish the assigned task more effectively?
  b How can you apply this knowledge to your relationships with your own family members?
  c How can you apply this knowledge to your relationships with your clients?

Simulation 2

The First Home Visit

This simulation requires seven players. Each player chooses a role, and reads the corresponding part description below. The roles available are:

  Player A Student nurse on her first home visit
  Player B Mrs. Smith, wife and mother
  Player C Robin Smith, 12
  Player D John Smith, 14, the identified patient
  Player E Timekeeper
  Player F Recorder
  Player G Coach

When players have read their role descriptions, they are to hold up a piece of paper in front of them or to wear a name tag telling others what role they are playing. After players have read their role descriptions, the coach has read each of the role cards, and each player has informed the timekeeper that he or she is ready, the timekeeper begins the simulation by saying, "Play out your roles."

Player A You are a student nurse about to make your first home visit. You are tense because you are not sure how the family will receive you. You are going to the home to assess the health needs of John, 14, who has diabetes, and to see what other health needs the family may have. The school nurse referred John to the agency because she thinks that John needs to learn more about diabetes and how to deal with it.

Player B You are Mrs. Smith, a wife and mother of two children, John and Robin. You know John does not follow his diet for diabetes, but right now you are more concerned with your thought that the student nurse has come to inspect your home and to make negative comments about your housekeeping and mothering skills. When the student nurse arrives, you let her knock several times, and then only open the door a crack; you do not allow her to enter your house right away. During the visit, you keep asking, "Why are you here, anyway?" "I don't need any help" and "I'm a good mother to John and Robin." You berate your father, Mr. Boyer, in the presence of both the nurse and the children ("What am I going to do with you; all you do is drink!") but, at the same time, you promote his drinking behavior ("Be quiet, dad, and I'll give you 5 dollars when the nurse leaves").

Player C You are Robin Smith, 12, the sister of John. He has diabetes, and you feel that your mother always gives him preferential treatment. Because of this, you are very loud and noisy and try to attract your mother's attention whenever she starts to talk to the student nurse about John. You interrupt John whenever he tries to talk, and ask the student nurse questions about her education, parents, home, and hobbies. You also bring the student nurse samples of things you have made in school for her to inspect and comment on.

Player D You are John, 14, the identified patient. You have diabetes, but try to pretend that you don't. You don't want to stick to your diet because the kids at school tease you about not being able to have a Coke and candy with them. You are aware that your mother is overly concerned about you, so you are distant toward her and always refer to her as "she." You answer the student nurse in words of one syllable whenever she asks you about your diabetes. Otherwise, you talk to the nurse and try to get her to be your ally. You wish you could be more outgoing like your sister Robin, but you don't let her know that you envy her; instead, you shout at her a lot and tell her to "Be quiet, Squirt" and "Get out of my way!"

Player E You are the timekeeper. You begin the simulation when all the other players have signalled you that they are ready to begin. You start the simulation and keep it going for 15 minutes. After 15 minutes, you call "Time," and then you lead the group discussion using the questions at the end of this simulation.

Player F You are the recorder. You may use the Family Observation and Assessment Guide to observe and record important elements of the interaction. When the timekeeper calls "Time," you are to use the information that you have collected to help the other players to answer the discussion questions. You may also refer to Chapters 5, 6, and 12.

Player G You are the coach. You are like the director of a play. You move around freely, coaching each of the players on what to say or to do if the action seems to be slowing down. For example, if the student nurse is too timid, tell her, "Say that more positively!" or if the mother is too hospitable, say, "Mrs. Smith, you're supposed to be suspicious of the student nurse," or if Robin is too quiet, tell her, "Start interrupting other people," or if Mr. Boyer is too cooperative, say, "Start bragging about or berating yourself for your drinking." In order to be an effective coach, you must read the parts of all the others players so that you can coach them to stay in their roles. During the discussion that follows this simulation, you can give examples your observations of how the other players could have been more effective during the interaction.

DISCUSSION QUESTIONS

1 Assessments
   a What can you say about the homeostatic devices in this family?
   b Was the Sick Role or the Different Role played by the identified patient in the simulation?
   c How well did the student nurse meet the family's need for orientation to the purpose of the visit?
   d What levels of anxiety did you observe in the family system and in the individuals as they interacted with each other?
   e Was conflict evident? What examples can you give to support your assessment?
   f Were there silences? What types of silences were they?
   g What coping devices did family members use? What coping devices did the student nurse use?
   h Were there evidences of dependency in this family?
   i At what phase of the grief process did the identified patient appear to be?
   j What examples of family interaction patterns did you observe? (Consider family norms, roles, effective and ineffective communication.)
   k What goals did the family have for treatment? Did the student nurse consider family goals, or even ask family members what they thought they needed help with?

l   What teaching/learning needs did this family have?

m What strengths did this family have?

n   How was the termination of the visit handled?

2   Interventions

a In what alternative ways could the student nurse have supported the Different Role for John?

b How could the student nurse have provided a more effective orientation to the purpose of the visit for this family?

c What could the student nurse have done to decrease the anxiety levels in herself and in others?

d How could the student nurse have dealt with the conflict that you observed?

e How could the student nurse have handled silences (if there were any) more effectively?

f Did the student nurse attempt to take away family (or individual) coping devices? Were her attempts effective? What changes would you suggest?

g How else could the student nurse have dealt with dependency?

h In what others ways could the student nurse have dealt with John's level of grief?

i What interventions could have been made to improve the effectiveness of family communication?

j How else might the student nurse have found out family goals for treatment?

k In what ways could the student nurse have begun to meet the family's needs for teaching/learning?

l How could the student have promoted family strengths?

m How could have the termination the visit been handled more effectively?

When you have answered the above questions, replay the simulation with different people taking different roles. Try to implement in this replay anything you may have learned from your discussion of assessment and intervention techniques.

Simulation 3

The Help-rejecting Family

This simulation requires four to seven players. The roles of timekeeper, recorder, and/or coach may be eliminated if no more than four people are available to carry out the simulation. Each player chooses a role, and reads the corresponding part description below. The roles are:

Player A Community health nurse
Player B Mrs. Galbrini, the identified patient
Player C Mr. Galbrini, husband of the identified patient
Player D Ms. Galbrini, 29, daughter who lives with her parents
Player E Timekeeper
Player F Recorder
Player G Coach

Players may identify themselves by wearing name tags. When players have read their role descriptions, the coach has read each of the role cards, and each player has informed the timekeeper that he or she is ready, the timekeeper begins the simulation by saying, "Play out your roles."

Player A You are a community health nurse who has visited the Galbrini home several times. No one has opened the door to you yet, although you have left several notes in the mailbox about wanting to talk with the family. You received a referral from the mobile chest x-ray unit that Mrs. Galbrini's x-ray was positive. You cannot understand why family members will not see you or accept your help, and you tell them this when you are finally admitted into their home.

Player B You are the identified patient, Mrs. Galbrini. You have had a chest x-ray recently, but only after hours of arguing with your daughter about the necessity of having one. You have had a persistent cough and have experienced increasing fatigue. You are afraid that you may have cancer and do not want to find out the results of the x-ray.

Player C You are Mr. Galbrini, husband of the identified patient. You are afraid that your wife is dying and you try to repress this idea by busying yourself with her care, by making all her decisions for her, and by acting like a tyrant in the presence of others.

Player D You are the unmarried daughter. You live at home with your parents. You are quiet and let your father think he has things in hand, although your salary pays the bills and you handle things when your father gets overemotional. You feel intimidated by him at times, but think that you could stand up for your rights with a little support.

Player E You are the timekeeper. You begin the simulation when all the other players have signalled you that they are ready to begin. You start the simulation and keep it going for 15 minutes. After 15 minutes, you call "Time," and then you lead the group discussion using the questions at the end of this simulation.

Player F You are the recorder. You may use the Family Observation and Assessment Guide to observe and record important elements of the interaction. When the timekeeper calls "Time," you are to use the information that you have collected to help the other players to answer the discussion questions. You may also refer to Chapters 5 and 6.

Player G You are the coach. You are like the director of a play. You move around freely, coaching each of the players on what to say or to do if the action seems to be slowing down. In order to be an effective coach, you must read the parts of all the other players so that you can coach them to stay in their roles.

DISCUSSION QUESTIONS

1 Assessments
   a What homeostatic devices did this family use?
   b Was the Sick Role or Different Role played by the identified patient in the simulation?
   c How well did the community health nurse meet the family's need for orientation to the purpose of the visit?
   d What is your reaction to the community health nurse's attempt to communicate with the Galbrinis by leaving notes for them?
   e What purpose could leaving such notes serve in establishing a relationship?
   f What levels of anxiety did you observe in the family system and in the individuals as they interacted with one another?
   g Was conflict evident? What examples can you give to support your assessment?
   h What coping devices did family members use?
   i What devices did the nurse use to cope with her feeling of being rejected?
   j What examples of family interaction patterns did you observe? (Consider family norms, roles, effective and ineffective communication.)
   k Did the nurse and the family reach a workable agreement about how they would work together?
   l What teaching/learning needs did this family have?
   m What strengths did this family have?
   n How was the termination of the visit handled?
2 Interventions
   a How could the nurse have been more supportive of this family's constructive coping devices?
   b How could the nurse have begun to increase effective communication among the members of this family?
   c How could the nurse have increased the separateness of family members?
   d How might the nurse have stated his or her intention to establish a working contract with this family?
   e How might the nurse continue to intervene with Ms. Galbrini?
   f How could have the termination of the visit been handled more effectively?

Simulation 4

Helping the Family to Clarify the Nursing Home Decision

This simulation requires five to eight players. Each player chooses a role, and reads the corresponding part description below. The roles available are:

Player A Community health nurse
Player B Mr. Roberts, husband of Mrs. Roberts
Player C Mrs. Roberts, wife of Mr. Roberts and daughter of Mrs. Henderson
Player D Mrs. Henderson, Mrs. Roberts's mother, the identified patient
Player E Mr. Henderson, son of Mrs. Henderson and brother of Mrs. Roberts
Player F Timekeeper (optional)
Player G Recorder (optional)
Player H Coach (optional)

Players may identify themselves by wearing name tags. When each player has informed the timekeeper that he or she is ready, the timekeeper begins the simulation by saying, "Play out your roles."

Player A You are the community health nurse. You have gathered the Roberts and Henderson family members together to discuss placing Mrs. Henderson in a nursing home. Although you have told everyone the purpose of the meeting, you anticipate some upset and denial. When the simulation starts, you begin by restating the purpose of the meeting.

Player B You are Mr. Roberts. You know that your wife is being pressured by other family members to place her mother in a nursing home. You feel confused about the whole thing and wish to stay out of it. When the simulation starts, you keep trying to make excuses to leave.

Player C You are Mrs. Roberts. You are quite upset and in conflict over this matter. You feel guilty and anxious about placing your mother in a nursing home while at the same time you are angry at your mother for being incontinent, demanding, and careless. You feel overwhelmed by the whole situation.

Player D You are Mrs. Henderson, candidate for the nursing home. You know that you are getting weaker and more forgetful. Last week you left the gas on in the kitchen and this week you were incontinent in the hallway twice. You are embarrassed and angry about what is happening to you, yet you are fearful of going to a nursing home. You are also angry with your daughter, Mrs. Roberts, because she scolds you and does not seem to understand what is happening to you.

Player E You are Mrs. Henderson's son. You complain openly about the poor care that your sister has been providing for your mother and you keep trying to make her feel guilty about sending your mother to a nursing home. On the other hand, you know that you could not handle having your mother in your home either, but you do not volunteer this information during the meeting unless you are asked.

Player F You are the timekeeper. You begin the simulation when all the other players have signalled you that they are ready to begin. You start the simulation and keep it going for 15 minutes. After 15 minutes, you call "Time," and then you lead the group discussion using the questions at the end of this simulation.

Player G You are the recorder. You may use the Family Observation and Assessment Guide to observe and record important elements of the interaction. When the timekeeper calls "Time," you are to use the information that you have collected to help the other players to answer the discussion questions. You may also refer to Chapters 5, 6, and 12.

Player H You are the coach. You are like the director of a play. You move around freely, coaching each of the players on what to say or to do if the action seems to be slowing down. In order to be an effective coach, you must read the parts of all the other players so that you can coach them to stay in their roles.

DISCUSSION QUESTIONS

Use Table 3-4, p. 42, to aid you in this discussion.

1 Assessments
   a What can you say about the homeostatic devices in this family?
   b How well did the community health nurse meet the family's need for orientation to the purpose of the meeting?
   c What levels of anxiety did you observe in the family system and in the individuals as they interacted with each other?
   d What examples of conflict did you observe?
   e What family alliances were present?
   f Did the nurse ally herself with anyone?
   g What coping devices did family members use?
   h What examples of family interaction patterns did you observe? (Consider family norms, roles, myths, and communication and decision-making patterns.)
   i What strengths did this family have?
   j Did the nurse elaborate the parts of the problem?
   k Did the nurse encourage the family to develop alternate solutions?

l   Did the nurse keep the discussion focused on the purpose of the meeting?
m   Did the nurse summarize frequently?
n   Did the nurse encourage the family to test solutions?
o   Did the nurse test for consensus of decision?
p   Did the nurse state aloud the decision that had been reached?
q   How was the termination of the visit handled?
2   Interventions
a   In what alternative ways could the nurse have handled family resistance to decision making?
b   In what alternative ways could the nurse have handled family conflict?
c   How could the nurse have supported constructive family coping devices?
d   How could the nurse have been more effective in helping the family to reach an effective decision?
e   How could have the termination of the visit been handled more effectively?

Simulation 5

Assessing Suicidal Potential

This simulation requires three to five players. Each player chooses a role, and reads the corresponding part description below. The roles available are:

Player A   Community health nurse
Player B   Mrs. Rogers, daughter of Mr. Condon
Player C   Mr. Condon, the identified patient
Player D   Timekeeper (optional)
Player E   Recorder (optional)

Players may wear name tags to identify themselves. When players have read their role descriptions and have informed the timekeeper that they are ready, the timekeeper begins the simulation by saying, "Play out your roles."

Player A   You are the community health nurse. You have come to the Rogers/Condon home at the request of Mrs. Rogers. You are there to evaluate the suicide potential of Mr. Condon and to formulate a plan of care based on this assessment. When the simulation begins you are entering the home. Structure the visit so that you can gather the information that you need to plan the client's care.

Player B   You are Mrs. Rogers. Your father, Mr. Condon, has made passing references to wanting to die and you are highly anxious and in conflict about how to handle this. You want the nurse to give you immediate help.

Player C You are the identified patient, Mr. Condon. You feel that you are a burden to your daughter and have withdrawn from her lately. You have been doing a lot of thinking about death recently. Your wife died 6 months ago and, although you did not react at the time, you have recently lost your appetite for food and your interest in living. You told your priest that you wish to rejoin your wife. Things are worse at night for you and that is the time when you dwell on rejoining your wife.

Player D You are the timekeeper. You begin the simulation when all the other players have signalled you that they are ready to begin. You start the simulation and keep it going for 15 minutes. After 15 minutes, you call "Time," and then you lead the group discussion using the questions at the end of this simulation.

Player E You are the recorder. You may use the Family Observation and Assessment Guide to observe and record important elements of the interaction. When the timekeeper calls "Time," you are to use the information that you have collected to help the other players to answer the discussion questions. You may also refer to Chapters 5, 6, and 12.

DISCUSSION QUESTIONS

1 Assessments
  a What observations did you make about this family's homeostatic devices?
  b What signs of failure to grieve did you observe?
  c What signs of depression did you observe?
  d How many high suicide predictors does Mr. Condon have?
  e How openly was the nurse able to deal with the topic of suicide?
  f Was conflict evident? What examples can you give to support your assessment?
  g What levels of anxiety did you observe in the family system and in the individuals as they interacted with each other?
  h What strengths did this family have?
  i How did the family's goals for treatment mesh with the nurse's goals?
  j What options did the nurse suggest to the family as ways in which to deal with suicidal thought and/or behavior?
  k Did the nurse place responsibility for Mr. Condon's suicidal behavior on the family?
2 Interventions
  a In what ways could the nurse have dealt with Mr. Condon's possible failure to grieve the loss of his wife?
  b How else might the nurse have assessed Mr. Condon's potential for suicide?
  c How could the nurse have built on existing family strengths to provide a support network for Mr. Condon?
  d What other ways could the nurse have intervened to decrease the client's potential for suicide?
  e What additional referrals might you make for this family?

Simulation 6

Practicing Behavior Rehearsal Techniques

This simulation requires two to four players. Each player chooses a role and reads the corresponding parts description below. The roles available are:

Player A Community health nurse
Player B Mrs. Thompson, 35, the identified patient who has multiple sclerosis
Player C Timekeeper (optional)
Player D Recorder (optional)

Players may identify themselves by wearing name tags. When players have read their role descriptions and have informed the timekeeper that they are ready, the timekeeper begins the simulation by saying, "Play out your roles."

Player A You are a community health nurse who has agreed to use behavioral rehearsal in order to assist Mrs. Thompson to overcome her anxiety about going to the doctor's office. When the simulation begins, you start to assist the client to practice the trip to the doctor's office. If necessary, refer to Chapter 8 for ideas about how to start.

Player B You are Mrs. Thompson, a young mother with multiple sclerosis, who is extremely anxious about going to the doctor's office. You are in a wheelchair and have difficulty transferring yourself, dealing with people who stare at you, and emptying your leg urinal. You are not sure that the community health nurse can help you, and at first you resist behavioral rehearsal saying that you will "never be able to visit the doctor anyway, so forget it!"

Player C You are the timekeeper. You begin the simulation when all the other players have signalled you that they are ready to begin. You start the simulation and keep it going for 15 minutes. After 15 minutes, you call "Time," and then you lead the group discussion using the questions at the end of this simulation.

Player D You are the recorder. When the timekeeper calls "Time," you are to use the information that you have collected to help the other players to answer the discussion questions.

DISCUSSION QUESTIONS

1 Assessments
    a How well did the community health nurse meet the client's need for orientation to the purpose of the visit?
    b At what stage of the grief process did the client seem to be?
    c What levels of anxiety did you observe in the individuals as they interacted with each other?
    d Was conflict evident? Give examples to support your assessment.
    e What coping devices did the client exhibit?
    f What strengths did the client display?
    g What goals did the client have for treatment?
    h What goals did the nurse have for treatment?
    i Did the nurse and client disagree over treatment goals? How?
    j What areas did the community health nurse omit in the behavioral rehearsal?
    k How was the termination of the visit handled?
2 Interventions
    a How else could the nurse have oriented the client to the purpose of the visit?
    b How might the nurse assist the client (and/or family) with unresolved grief?
    c What else could the nurse have done to reduce the client's anxiety?
    d How else might the community health nurse have decreased the client's conflict over going to the doctor's office?
    e How else might the nurse have supported the client's healthy coping devices?
    f If you were the community health nurse, how would you draw up a behavioral contract with this client?
    g What would you add to or delete from the behavioral rehearsal used by the nurse?
    h How else might the termination of the visit have been handled?

Simulation 7

Conducting a Family Session with Potentially Abusing Parents

This simulation requires three to five players. Each player chooses a role, and reads the corresponding part description below. The roles available are:

Player A Nick DeGrasso, 38
Player B Ellen DeGrasso, 34, wife and new mother, the identified patient

Player C Community health nurse
Player D Timekeeper (optional)
Player E Recorder (optional)

When players have read their role descriptions and have informed the timekeeper that they are ready, the timekeeper begins the simulation by saying, "Play out your roles."

Player A You are Nick DeGrasso, a father for the first time. You have recently lost your job and you are frustrated with your life situation. You are a physical person who often gets into fist fights. You have hit your wife on occasion, but do not readily admit to this.

Player B You are Ellen DeGrasso. You got pregnant by mistake and have produced a female infant who cries a lot, who has constant diaper rash, and whom you are afraid to hold or to handle. Your mother used to hit you whenever she thought you misbehaved, and you are afraid that something terrible is going to happen to your baby.

Player C You are the community health nurse who is evaluating this family. At the start of the simulation, you are beginning to interview Nick and Ellen in order to formulate treatment goals.

Player D You are the timekeeper. You begin the simulation when all players have signalled you that they are ready to begin. You start the simulation and keep it going for 15 minutes. After 15 minutes, you call "Time," and then lead the group discussion using the questions at the end of this simulation.

Player E You are the recorder. You may use the Family Observation and Assessment Guide to observe and record important elements of the interaction. When the timekeeper calls "Time," you are to use the information that you have collected to help the other players to answer the discussion questions. You may also refer to Chapters 4, 5, and 6.

DISCUSSION QUESTIONS

1 Assessments
   a What observations did you make about the homeostatic devices in this family?
   b Were roles complementary or symmetrical?
   c How well did the nurse meet the marital pair's need for orientation to the purpose of the visit?

d What levels of anxiety did you observe in the family system and in the individuals as they interacted with each other? Give examples.
e Was conflict noted? Give examples.
f What coping devices were used?
g What examples of family interaction patterns did you observe?
h What goals did the family have for treatment?
i What goals did the nurse have for treatment?
j What disparity was there in the family's and in the nurse's goals?
k What strengths did the family have?
l What questions to assess the family's potential for child abuse did the nurse fail to ask?
m Which of the following techniques did the community health nurse use? (Refer to Chapter 5 if necessary.)

Establishing rapport
Example:

Using the family's language
Example:

Encouraging democratic values
Example:

Refraining from blaming or siding with family members
Example:

Modeling clear, effective communication
Example:

Eliciting alternate strategies for dealing with health problems
Example:

Teaching family members how to disagree constructively
Example:

Teaching family members how to contract with one another
Example:

2 Interventions
  a How else could the community health nurse have stated the purpose of the visit?
  b What else could the community health nurse have done to decrease anxiety levels?
  c What patterns of family interaction might the nurse choose to strengthen or change?
  d How could the nurse have supported constructive family coping devices?
  e If you were the community health nurse, how would you formulate a treatment contract with this family?
  f What additional assessment questions would you ask to judge this family's potential for abuse? (Refer to Chapter 4.)
  g What different communication techniques would you have used? Formulate specific comments or actions.
  h How else would you have handled the termination of the visit?
  i Would you make any referrals for this family? If so, to whom?

Answer Key

ANSWERS TO CHAPTER 1 REVIEW

Multiple-Choice Questions

1 a, b   **2** a, b, c

Listing

how successful usual coping devices are; the meaning of the symptoms to the sick person; the meaning ascribed to the symptoms by the sociocultural group; the number and persistence of symptoms; the degree of disruption of life-style

ANSWERS TO CHAPTER 2 REVIEW

Definition

unexplained feeling of discomfort learned in relation to others

Listing

1 the unexpected; the unfamiliar; the embarrassing; having to perform when unsure of oneself; unmet needs

2 mild; moderate; severe; panic

3 a Identify the feeling. Find out what preceded the feeling and how anxiety is relieved. Find a factor common to anxiety-provoking situations. Examine alternate ways to deal with anxiety. Use the prepractice exercises.

 b Remain present. Reduce sensory input. Use short and concise orienting statements.

Matching Terms

1 d   **2** a, c, e   **3** b

ANSWERS TO CHAPTER 3 REVIEW

Multiple-Choice Questions

1 a, b, d   **2** b, d

Definition

I can only be responsible for structuring health care situations when I am with the client, and, even then, he or she has the option of either working toward or not working toward my goals.

ANSWERS TO CHAPTER 4 REVIEW

Multiple-Choice Questions

1 c   **2** a, c, d

Listing

1 structured tasks; role-playing situations; firm insistence and acceptance of anger; assessment of your own need to be liked

2 Examine your own anxiety or guilt. Bring the suicidal person's behavior out into the open and discuss it. Place responsibility for the client's behavior on his or her family and friends. Suggest options to the family.

Matching Terms

1 d   **2** a   **3** b   **4** c

ANSWERS TO CHAPTER 5 REVIEW

Listing

Members are confident about their ability to relate to one another. Communication is clear and direct and feedback is asked for and responded to. Disagreement can occur without belittlement. Others are treated as having the potential for being masterful, sexual people. Tasks can be accomplished without resentment.

Matching Terms

1 b   2 d   3 e   4 c   5 a

ANSWERS TO CHAPTER 6 REVIEW

Multiple-Choice Questions

1 b, d

Listing

Plan visits to the family to establish person-to-person relationships with each member. Visit the family during periods of emotional upset, being careful not to form triangles.

Matching Terms

1 d   2 b   3 c   4 a

ANSWERS TO CHAPTER 7 REVIEW

Multiple-Choice Questions

1 a, d   2 a, c, e

Listing

1 learned, reinforced response to depression, anxiety, and negative interpersonal relationships; symptom of family disorganization
2 persecutor; patsy; connection; rescuer
3 Collect baseline data via food intake record. Chart weight daily on graph paper. Learn how to visualize ideal self. Set realistic goals. Begin exercise program. List enjoyed activities. Structure eating environment to make it difficult to overeat. Reward self for meeting goals and punish self when goals are not met.

ANSWERS TO CHAPTER 8 REVIEW

Multiple-Choice Questions

1 b, d

Matching Terms

1 e   2 g   3 b   4 d   5 a   6 f   7 c

ANSWERS TO CHAPTER 9 REVIEW

Listing

1 who the community is; how needs are met; how deviance and disturbance are handled; how identities are developed; how community functions are accomplished
2 What other factors in the system will be affected as a result of the change? What forces are operating to inhibit change? What information or experiences must precede the change? What new procedures or experiences will need to be developed as a result of the change? Who is likely to suffer from the change? How will power, influence, custom, or life-style be affected by the change? How aware is the client of the need for change or of its purpose? Is the client sufficiently involved in planning for the change? What is the relationship between the change agent and the client? What past relationships between the change agent (or agency) and the client might be influencing resistance now? How open has the client been to the introduction of change in the past?
3 decreasing anxiety; channeling conflict into constructive discussion; agreeing to modify goals; using appropriate timing; projecting confidence that change can occur; providing rewards for change; working with system leaders; and proving credibility as a change agent

ANSWERS TO CHAPTER 10 REVIEW

Definition

verbatim, sequential report of the client's verbal and nonverbal communication, of the nurse's verbal and nonverbal communication, and of the nurse's analysis, evaluation, and speculations about the communications

Matching Terms

1 d   2 c   3 e   4 a   5 b

ANSWERS TO CHAPTER 11 REVIEW

Listing

1 orientation; anxiety; suicidal potential; coping devices; conflict; communication; grief/loss/depression; dependency/problem solving; family interaction; termination of nurse-client relationship
2 client's view of treatment; client's goals for treatment; client's self-view; recent changes or losses; physical complaints; other therapies; feeling difficulties; thought difficulties; action difficulties; communication difficulties; relationships with others; developmental difficulties; coping devices and strengths; goals for the future

ANSWERS TO CHAPTER 12 REVIEW

Listing

who is present; seating arrangement; anxiety levels; family norms; critical events; roles; functional and dysfunctional family relationships; leadership; disruptions; general atmosphere; phases of interaction

ANSWERS TO CHAPTER 13 REVIEW

Definition

a recurrent happening or message

Listing

1 feeling increasingly uncomfortable when working with a client
2 Themes are clearer indicants of how clients view themselves and others than isolated phrases or answers are; they give the nurse clues about his or her own blind spots and reactions to patients.
3 "I don't have that many problems!" "I don't need psychotherapy." "Perhaps the consultant can just take over the case." "I must not be very competent if I need consultation." "I don't have any psychiatric clients, so why would I need mental health nursing consultation?" "I don't have time to sit down with a consultant." "Consultants may know a lot of theory, but they don't know much about actually working with clients."

Index